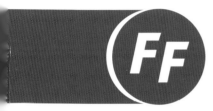

FAST FACTS

Brain Tumors

Indispensable
Guides to
Clinical
Practice

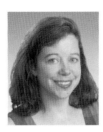

Lauren E Abrey

Attending Neurologist
Department of Neurology
Memorial Sloan–Kettering Cancer Center
New York, NY, USA

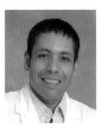

Warren P Mason

Staff Physician
Department of Medical Oncology and Hematology
Pencer Brain Tumor Centre
Princess Margaret Hospital
Toronto, Ontario, Canada

This book is as balanced and as practical as we can make it. Ideas for improvement are always welcome: feedback@fastfactsbooks.com

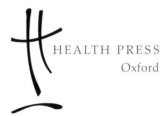

HEALTH PRESS
Oxford

Fast Facts – Brain Tumors
First published December 2003

Text © 2003 Lauren E Abrey, Warren P Mason

© 2003 in this edition Health Press Limited
Health Press Limited, Elizabeth House, Queen Street, Abingdon,
Oxford OX14 3JR, UK
Tel: +44 (0)1235 523233
Fax: +44 (0)1235 523238

Book orders can be placed by telephone or via the website.
For regional distributors or to order via the website, please go to:
www.fastfacts.com
For telephone orders, please call 01752 202301 (UK) or
1 800 538 1287 (North America, toll free).

Fast Facts is a trademark of Health Press Limited.

The publisher and the authors have made every effort to ensure the
accuracy of this book, but cannot accept responsibility for any errors or
omissions.

Registered names, trademarks, etc. used in this book, even when not
marked as such, are not to be considered unprotected by law.

A CIP catalogue record for this title is available from the British Library.

ISBN 1-903734-43-6

Abrey LE (Lauren)
Fast Facts – Brain Tumors/
Lauren E Abrey, Warren P Mason

Typesetting and page layout by Zed, Oxford, UK.
Printed by Fine Print (Services) Ltd, Oxford, UK.

Printed with vegetable inks on fully biodegradable and
recyclable paper manufactured from sustainable forests.

Low emissions
during production

Low
chlorine

Sustainable
forests

Introduction

The term 'brain tumor' encompasses a wide range of tumor types, including malignant tumors arising from the brain parenchyma, low-grade tumors arising from the meninges or pituitary gland, and a variety of other rare tumors. The approach to managing patients with these various types of brain tumors is truly multidisciplinary, involving primary care physicians, neurologists, radiologists, neurosurgeons, pathologists, radiation oncologists and neuro-oncologists. Provision of optimal care for an individual patient requires adequate input from each specialty in order to synthesize an appropriate diagnostic and therapeutic plan.

Advances in radiology and pathology allow more precise and detailed diagnoses than ever before. Similarly, developments in molecular biology and imaging techniques are constantly improving available diagnostic modalities. Furthermore, advances in neurosurgical techniques enable us to operate on tumors previously considered inoperable, and novel delivery systems allow various treatments to reach tumors otherwise protected by the blood–brain barrier. Increasingly, chemotherapy is being used successfully to treat patients with primary brain tumors, and the development of numerous biological agents, such as anti-angiogenic agents, holds great promise for the future. In addition, developments in computer planning and radiobiology have resulted in improvements in the precision with which radiation oncologists can treat intracranial tumors.

In this book, we have attempted to summarize the salient features of each of the various brain tumors and treatment modalities in a way that will be useful to the practicing clinician. Perhaps the most important message is that there are currently a variety of effective therapies available to a patient diagnosed with a brain tumor. Therefore, it is critically important to give careful thought to the best initial approach for an individual patient in order to achieve the best overall outcome, both in terms of survival and quality of life.

1 Classification and epidemiology

Classification

Intracranial tumors can be classified in several different ways. The most fundamental differentiation is between primary intracranial lesions and metastatic tumors. Primary tumors can be further subdivided according to whether they arise from the brain parenchyma, meninges, pituitary region, pineal region or skull base.

Neurological symptoms and neuroimaging provide information about tumor location, which is useful in developing a differential diagnosis (Table 1.1). However, definitive diagnosis of primary brain tumors is based on the cell of origin and requires histopathological assessment, the gold standard for diagnosis. Table 1.2 shows the World Health Organization (WHO) classification of these tumors.

The majority of intracranial tumors arise from the brain parenchyma, primarily from glial cells (astrocytes or oligodendrocytes). Primary neuronal tumors are uncommon. Meningeal tumors are the second most common type of intracranial tumor. Tumors also arise from a variety of other cell types, including some not ordinarily found in the brain, such as germ cells, lymphocytes and rests of embryonic tissues (Figure 1.1).

Incidence and epidemiology

Brain metastases are much more common than primary intracranial tumors. Approximately 170 000 people in the USA are diagnosed with brain metastases every year, while 39 550 are diagnosed with a primary benign or malignant brain tumor. More than 13 000 die each year as a result of a primary malignant brain tumor. In children and men aged 20–39 years, brain tumors are the second leading cause of cancer-related death in the USA.

Data from several studies suggest an increase in the incidence of both primary brain tumors, particularly primary central nervous system (CNS) lymphoma, and brain metastases since the 1970s. This may be

TABLE 1.1

Brain tumor classification by location

Cerebral hemisphere

- Gliomas
- Primary central nervous system lymphoma
- Meningioma
- Ependymoma
- Metastases

Intraventricular

- Ependymoma/ subependymoma
- Subependymal giant cell astrocytoma (tuberous sclerosis)
- Central neurocytoma
- Colloid cyst of the third ventricle
- Meningioma
- Choroid plexus papilloma/carcinoma

Cerebellum

- Medulloblastoma
- Hemangioblastoma
- Dermoid/epidermoid tumor
- Pilocytic astrocytoma
- Astrocytoma
- Dysplastic gangliocytoma (Lhermitte–Duclos disease)
- Metastases

Cerebellopontine angle

- Vestibular schwannoma
- Meningioma
- Epidermoid
- Choroid plexus papilloma
- Metastases

Sellar region

- Pituitary adenoma
- Germ cell tumor
- Craniopharyngioma
- Meningioma
- Rathke cleft cyst
- Lymphoma
- Metastases

Pineal region

- Pineal parenchymal tumor
- Germ cell tumor
- Meningioma
- Tectal glioma
- Dermoid/epidermoid tumor

Skull base

- Meningioma
- Cranial nerve schwannoma
- Paraganglioma
- Chordoma
- Esthesioneuroblastoma
- Primary sarcoma or carcinoma
- Metastases

TABLE 1.2

Histological classification of brain tumors

Neuroepithelial tumors

Astrocytic tumors

- Pilocytic astrocytoma (WHO grade I)
- Diffuse astrocytoma (WHO grade II)
- Anaplastic astrocytoma (WHO grade III)
- Glioblastoma multiforme (WHO grade IV)
- Pleomorphic xanthoastrocytoma
- Subependymal giant cell astrocytoma

Oligodendroglial tumors

- Oligodendroglioma, low-grade or anaplastic

Ependymal tumors

- Ependymoma, low-grade or anaplastic
- Myxopapillary ependymoma
- Subependymoma

Choroid plexus tumors

- Choroid plexus papilloma
- Choroid plexus carcinoma

Neuronal/mixed glial–neuronal tumors

- Gangliocytoma
- Ganglioglioma
- Dysembryoplastic neuroepithelial tumor
- Central neurocytoma

Pineal parenchymal tumors

- Pineocytoma
- Pineal parenchymal tumor of intermediate differentiation
- Pineoblastoma

Embryonal tumors

- Medulloblastoma
- Primitive neuroectodermal tumor (PNET)
- Atypical teratoid/rhabdoid tumor

Tumors of cranial nerves

- Schwannoma
- Neurofibroma
- Malignant peripheral nerve sheath tumor

Meningeal tumors

- Meningioma
- Hemangiopericytoma
- Hemangioblastoma
- Melanocytoma

Germ cell tumors

- Germinoma
- Embryonal carcinoma
- Yolk sac tumor (endodermal sinus tumor)
- Choriocarcinoma
- Teratoma, mature or immature

(CONTINUED)

TABLE 1.2 (CONTINUED)

Primary CNS lymphoma

Tumors of the sellar region
- Pituitary adenoma – not included in WHO CNS tumors
- Craniopharyngioma
- Granular cell tumor

Cysts and tumor-like lesions – not included in WHO CNS tumors
- Rathke cleft cysts
- Epidermoid cyst
- Dermoid cyst
- Colloid cyst of the third ventricle

Metastatic tumors – not included in WHO CNS tumors

Adapted from the WHO classification of brain tumors

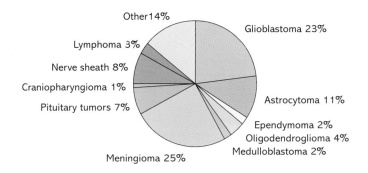

Figure 1.1 Relative distribution of primary brain tumors by histology.

partly due to a true increase in incidence, but is also a consequence of greater access to imaging and improved neuroimaging techniques.

Epidemiological studies of brain tumors are limited and often flawed as a result of ascertainment bias, small sample size and retrospective design. The best data suggest an annual incidence for primary brain tumors of 10–19/100 000 person-years. The incidence of primary brain tumors varies by sex, race, age and geography. Men have a higher risk than women of developing most brain tumors, with the exception of meningiomas. Similarly, brain tumors are more common in Caucasians than other ethnic groups, with the exception of meningiomas and pituitary adenomas.

To date, only two unequivocal risk factors have been identified: ionizing radiation and immune suppression. Numerous other risk factors have been reported (Table 1.3) but the studies are generally small and their findings have not been reproduced.

An increasing number of molecular genetic alterations have been described in association with particular primary brain tumors (Table 1.4). In the majority of patients, it is likely that some combination of genetic and environmental factors leads to the development of a brain tumor.

Developments in molecular biology, genomics and proteomics are resulting in an exponential increase in our knowledge about all types of brain tumors, and should lead to the development of novel therapeutic strategies.

TABLE 1.3

Possible risk factors for brain tumors

- Electromagnetic fields
- Diet
  - N-nitroso compounds
  - Aspartame
  - Maternal alcohol consumption
- Occupation
  - Petroleum industry
  - Pesticide or chemical exposure
- Head trauma
- Household chemicals
- Infection
  - Tuberculosis
  - Varicella zoster
  - Simian virus 40 infection

TABLE 1.4

Molecular genetic abnormalities associated with brain tumors

Tumor type	Genetic abnormality	Implication
High-grade glioma	$p53$ pathway – $p53$ mutation – $MDM2$ over-expression – $p14^{ARF}$ loss	Loss of normal apoptosis with cellular injury
	$EGFR$ amplification	Promotes cell growth, blocks cell death
	$PTEN$ mutation	Important in phosphatase pathways
	RB pathway – RB loss – $CDK4$ amplification – $p16^{INK4A}$ deletion	Allows for uncontrolled cell growth
Pilocytic astrocytoma	$17q$ loss/$NF1$ mutation	Enhanced cellular motility and attachment Associated with neurofibromatosis type 1
Medulloblastoma*	$17p$ loss/$17q$ gain	May be associated with poor prognosis
	N-myc, C-myc amplification	May be associated with poor prognosis
Pituitary adenoma	$11q$ loss	Associated with MEN-1 syndrome
Meningioma	$22q$ LOH/$NF2$ inactivation	Associated with neurofibromatosis type 2

*May be seen in association with Li-Fraumeni, Gorlin, blue rubber bleb nevus and Turcot syndromes.

ARF, alternative reading frame (a tumor suppressor gene product that sensitizes cells to apoptosis); EGFR, epidermal growth factor receptor; MDM2, mouse double minute 2 gene; PTEN, phosphate and tensin analog deleted from chromosome 10; RB, retinoblastoma gene; CDK, cyclin-dependent kinase; INK4A, one of a family of cyclin-dependent kinase inhibitors; NF1, neurofibromatosis-1 gene; NF2, neurofibromatosis-2 gene; LOH, loss of heterozygosity.

Key points – classification and epidemiology

- Primary brain tumors and metastases have both been diagnosed with increasing frequency over the past few decades. This may reflect a true increase in incidence, but improved neuroimaging techniques and greater access to imaging account for a portion of this increase.
- Environmental risk factors for the development of brain tumors are poorly understood and probably over-reported.
- Developments in molecular biology, genomics and proteomics are resulting in an exponential increase in our knowledge about all types of brain tumors.

Key references

Central Brain Tumor Registry of the United States. *Statistical Report: Primary Brain Tumors in the United States, 1995–1999.* Chicago, IL: Central Brain Tumor Registry of the United States, 2002.

Kleihues P, Cavanee WK. *World Health Organization Classification of Tumours: Tumours of the Nervous System – Pathology and Genetics.* Lyon, France: IRAC Press, 2000.

Wrensch M, Minn Y, Chew T et al. Epidemiology of primary brain tumors: current concepts and review of the literature. *Neuro-oncol* 2002; 4:278–99.

Neurological signs and symptoms

Patients with brain tumors typically develop neurological signs and symptoms over a period of weeks to months. Some will have an abrupt onset of signs and symptoms similar to that seen in patients with a cerebrovascular infarct. Occasionally, however, patients will have signs or symptoms, such as a chronic seizure disorder, for years prior to the diagnosis of a low-grade tumor.

Symptoms and signs may result from increased intracranial pressure, tumor invasion, obstructive hydrocephalus, tumor secretions or secondary cerebral ischemia. Initial symptoms are often vague and non-specific (Table 2.1). The neurological examination may be normal. Hence, a high index of suspicion is necessary so that no clinical clues are disregarded.

Some typical misleading scenarios include a sudden or insidious change in personality or mood that is misdiagnosed as depression but is refractory to therapy, or an unexplained change in a patient's usual headache pattern or the development of new headaches in an atypical age group (young children or older adults).

The various neurological symptoms and signs caused by brain tumors may be generalized, localizing or falsely localizing.

TABLE 2.1

Common signs and symptoms of a brain tumor

• None	• Seizures
• Headache	• Focal weakness
• Nausea/vomiting	• Difficulty walking
• Confusion	• Double vision
• Personality change	• Visual loss
• Memory loss	• Tinnitus

Headache is the most common symptom of a brain tumor. Typically, the headache is non-specific and occurs equally in patients with and without increased intracranial pressure. Since headache is also the most common neurological complaint in the general population, it is important to note specific features of a patient's headache, as these can assist the diagnostic evaluation. Features that should increase suspicion of a tumor include:
- daily headache on waking that improves over a short interval of time
- new headache in a middle-aged or older person
- change in pattern, character or severity of a chronic headache
- exacerbation of headache by coughing, sneezing, bending, head movement or exertion
- headache accompanied by other neurological symptoms
- acute headache followed by vomiting.

Although headache is the most common symptom of a brain tumor, many patients do not have a headache.

Other generalized signs and symptoms. Poorly described dizziness and tinnitus are common complaints. Papilledema may be an incidental finding on ophthalmologic examination.

Transient elevations in intracranial pressure may lead to a variety of confusing neurological features, including headache, visual loss, change in level of consciousness, loss of muscle tone, itching, shivering, yawning and hiccups. These events, called plateau waves, are often precipitated by change in position and may be mistaken for a seizure.

Localizing and falsely localizing features. The most common localizing sign of a brain tumor is seizure; patients typically have focal seizures with or without secondary generalization. Other focal findings depend on the site of the lesion and include hemiparesis, aphasia, visual field loss and sensory disturbance (Table 2.2). Falsely localizing signs seen with increased intracranial pressure include: cranial nerve I, III, IV, VI or VIII abnormality, ipsilateral hemiparesis and ataxia (Table 2.3).

Seizures occur in about one-third of patients; they are often the initial and only symptom. Up to 20% of adults with new onset seizures will have an underlying brain tumor. Seizures are more common in

TABLE 2.2

Common findings on examining patients with brain tumors

- None
- Abnormal mental status
- Papilledema
- Cranial neuropathy
- Hemiparesis
- Sensory loss
- Ataxia

TABLE 2.3

False localizing symptoms and signs in patients with brain tumors

- Anosmia
- Diplopia (usually cranial nerve VI palsy)
- Tinnitus
- Ipsilateral hemiparesis
- Ipsilateral gaze paresis
- Cortical blindness
- Nuchal rigidity

low-grade than high-grade tumors. Focal seizures are common in situations where the tumor compresses cortex, especially adjacent to the motor strip. Patients with an abrupt or unexplained change in level of function may have non-convulsive status epilepticus; this is not always accompanied by a demonstrable change in level of consciousness and should be evaluated by an EEG.

Imaging modalities

Magnetic resonance imaging. Gadolinium-enhanced magnetic resonance imaging (MRI) is the gold standard for the imaging of brain tumors. This imaging technique gives the best anatomic detail of the brain and other intracranial structures. Specific signal characteristics often allow the radiologist to predict the histological diagnosis (Table 2.4).

Perfusion magnetic resonance images give an indication of tumor vascularity and may be a reliable marker of tumor grade. Magnetic resonance spectroscopy allows the measurement of biochemical spectra in a region of interest; certain patterns of change may correlate with tumor histology or grade (Figures 2.1 and 2.2, Table 2.5). Functional MRI allows areas of brain function to be mapped. This may be useful

TABLE 2.4

Magnetic resonance imaging characteristics of selected central nervous system tumors

	T2	T1	Gd-enhancement
Low-grade glioma	Hyperintense	Hypointense	±, patchy
High-grade glioma	Hyperintense	Hypointense	+, irregular, peripheral
PCNSL	Hyperintense	Hyperintense	+, uniform, dense
Metastasis	Variable	Mixed	+, ring like
Meningioma	Iso-intense to hypointense	Iso-intense to hyperintense	+

Gd, gadolinium; PCNSL, primary central nervous system lymphoma

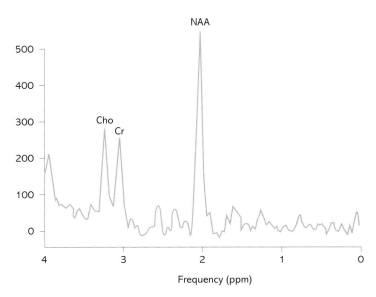

Figure 2.1 Magnetic resonance spectroscopy of normal brain tissue. NAA, N-acetyl aspartate (neuronal and axonal marker) 2 ppm; Cho, choline (signifying cellular membrane turnover) 3.2 ppm; Cr, creatine (energy metabolism) 3 ppm. Peaks that may be seen in abnormal tissues include: myo-inositol (signifying protein C activation) 3.6 ppm, lactate (anaerobic metabolism) 1.3 ppm and lipid (necrosis) 0.9 ppm.

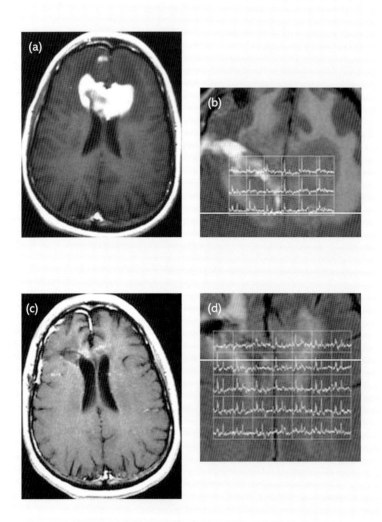

Figure 2.2 (a) Gadolinium-enhanced T1-weighted axial MRI and
(b) corresponding magnetic resonance spectroscopy image of a patient with
primary CNS lymphoma at diagnosis. (c) Gadolinium-enhanced T1-weighted
axial MRI and (d) magnetic resonance spectroscopy image of the same patient
following treatment with chemotherapy. These images demonstrate normalization
of the magnetic resonance spectra corresponding with the radiographic response
to treatment.

TABLE 2.5

Magnetic resonance spectroscopy changes in brain tumors

High-grade tumors

- Elevated choline to N-acetyl aspartate ratio
- Decreased to absent N-acetyl aspartate
- Decreased myo-inositol
- Lipid present
- Lactate variable

Low-grade tumors

- Slight increase in choline
- Slight decrease N-acetyl aspartate
- Increased myo-inositol
- No lipid

for presurgical planning to allow maximal resection while sparing critical areas of neurological function.

Magnetic resonance spectroscopy may also be useful in assessing the response to newer therapies, particularly targeted molecular strategies that may be cytostatic.

Computerized tomography (CT) is superior to MRI for visualizing calcification and may be useful in certain types of tumor, such as meningiomas or oligodendrogliomas, that are prone to calcification. CT scanning may also be helpful in determining the extent of bony destruction or hyperostosis related to tumor growth. Patients with a medical contraindication for MRI (e.g. cardiac pacemaker, ferromagnetic foreign body) should be imaged with CT.

Positron emission tomography (PET) is a nuclear medicine study that provides metabolic tumor imaging. A variety of different substances can be labeled with a positron-emitting isotope:

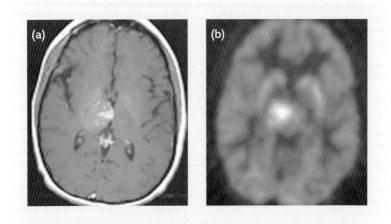

Figure 2.3 Gadolinium-enhanced T1-weighted axial MRI and corresponding 18-fluoro-2-deoxyglucose PET imaging of a thalamic glioma. This image was used to guide stereotactic biopsy of this lesion.

18-fluoro-2-deoxyglucose, the most common isotope, images glucose metabolism; 11-carbon-methionine, an amino acid, images DNA metabolism. Uptake is increased in proportion with tumor grade.

PET scans are clinically useful in guiding stereotactic needle biopsy (Figure 2.3), or differentiating radiation necrosis from recurrent tumor. In the future, they may be important in determining response to newer classes of antitumor drugs such as anti-angiogenic agents.

Single photon emission computed tomography (SPECT) is a less technically demanding nuclear medicine image that is more widely available than PET. SPECT may be useful in differentiating tumor from radiation necrosis, and has been used extensively to differentiate between tumor and infection in HIV-positive patients.

Pathology
Definitive histopathologic diagnosis is essential before administering specific antitumor therapy. The only exception is diffuse pontine glioma, as this diagnosis can usually be made on the basis of the

characteristic MRI appearance and the risk of neurological injury subsequent to biopsy outweighs any benefit.

A neuropathologist should review all specimens; ideally, an intraoperative frozen section should be obtained and as large a sample as possible submitted for final review. Furthermore, the pathologist should be apprised of:

- the patient's age and clinical presentation
- the radiographic appearance of the tumor
- prior therapy, including preoperative interventions such as embolization that may cause focal necrosis.

These factors may be critical in the interpretation of pathological findings and guide the selection of appropriate immunohistochemical stains (Table 2.6) or other specialized studies (e.g. electron microscopy).

Clinical correlation is critical to the interpretation of both neuroimaging and pathology. Ideally, the clinician should review images and pathology information directly with the radiologist and neuropathologist.

TABLE 2.6

Immunoreactivity of selected brain tumors

	EMA	CK	S-100	CEA	LCA	Vimentin	GFAP
Glioma	−	+	+	−	−	+	+
PCNSL	−	−	−	−	+	±	−
Metastasis	+	+	±	±	−	±	−
Meningioma	+	±	±	±	−	+	−
Medulloblastoma	−	−	±	−	−	±	±
Choroid plexus tumor	±	±	+	±	−	+	±
Schwannoma	±	−	+	−	−	+	±

PCNSL, primary central nervous system lymphoma; EMA, epithelial membrane antigen; CK, creatine kinase; S-100, one of a family of proteins; CEA, carcinoembryonic antigen; LCA, leukocyte common antigen; GFAP, glial fibrillary acidic protein

Key points – diagnosis

- Initial symptoms and signs of a brain tumor are often vague or non-specific; many patients will have a normal neurological examination.
- Headache, the most common symptom of a brain tumor, is also the most common neurological complaint in the general population. Therefore, attention to specific features of a patient's headache should guide the clinician's index of suspicion and diagnostic evaluation.
- Seizures occur in one-third of patients and any adult with new onset seizures should be evaluated for an underlying brain tumor.
- Although neuroimaging may suggest a specific diagnosis, tissue should be obtained for pathological review in all patients before instituting any therapy. The only exception to this rule is the patient with a typical infiltrating pontine glioma, where the risks of surgery outweigh the benefit.
- Ideally, the clinician should review images and pathology information directly with the radiologist and neuropathologist.
- Improvements in neuro-imaging may be most useful in assessing response to newer therapies, particularly targeted molecular strategies that may be cytostatic.

Key references

Burger PC, Scheithauer BW. *Atlas of Tumor Pathology: Tumors of the Central Nervous System.* Washington, DC: Armed Forces Institute of Pathology, 1994.

Dowling C, Bollen AW, Noworolski SM et al. Preoperative proton MR spectroscopic imaging of brain tumors: correlation with histopathologic analysis of resection specimens. *Am J Neuroradiol* 2001; 22:604–12.

Forsyth PA, Posner JB. Headaches in patients with brain tumors: a study of 111 patients. *Neurology* 1993;43: 1678–83.

Hustinx R, Alavi A. SPECT and PET imaging of brain tumors. *Neuroimaging Clin N Am* 1999; 9:751–66.

Kremer S, Grand S, Remy C et al. Cerebral blood volume mapping by MR imaging in the initial evaluation of brain tumors. *J Neuroradiol* 2002; 29:105–13.

Leclerc X, Huisman TA, Sorensen AG. The potential of proton magnetic resonance spectroscopy (1H-MRS) in the diagnosis and management of patients with brain tumors. *Curr Opin Oncol* 2002; 14:292–8.

Nelson SJ. Analysis of volume MRI and MR spectroscopic imaging data for the evaluation of patients with brain tumors. *Magn Reson Med* 2001;46:228–39.

Provenzale JM, Wang GR, Brenner T et al. Comparison of permeability in high-grade and low-grade brain tumors using dynamic susceptibility contrast MR imaging. *Am J Roentgenol* 2002;178:711–16.

Roberts HC, Roberts TP, Bollen AW et al. Correlation of microvascular permeability derived from dynamic contrast-enhanced MR imaging with histologic grade and tumor labeling index: a study in human brain tumors. *Acad Radiol* 2001;8:384–91.

Snyder H, Robinson K, Shah D et al. Signs and symptoms of patients with brain tumors presenting to the emergency department. *J Emerg Med* 1993;11:253–8.

Surgery

The main reasons for surgical intervention in patients with brain tumors are:

- to obtain tissue for accurate pathological diagnosis
- to relieve symptoms and improve outcome by maximal surgical resection.

The past decades have brought about remarkable advances in the technical aspects of tumor removal. One such advance has been the routine use of cortical mapping and stereotactic volumetric resections. Other improvements have been seen in the area of surgical equipment, including robotics, lasers and ultrasonic aspirators. Together, these developments have improved the surgeon's ability to perform radical resection of brain tumors, many of which had previously been considered inoperable.

The surgeon's role has always been central in the management of patients with brain tumors, and recent studies have demonstrated a favorable association between cytoreductive surgery and prognosis for a variety of brain neoplasms, including brain metastases and low- and high-grade gliomas.

Perioperative assessment. The principal components of preoperative assessment of patients with brain tumor are the history, physical examination and imaging. The history and physical examination provide valuable information regarding the most likely diagnosis, and the potential role and risks of surgery. Following the clinical assessment, imaging plays a crucial role in surgical planning.

The most commonly used preoperative imaging modalities are magnetic resonance imaging (MRI) and computerized tomography (CT). MRI provides superior images of tumor location and extent, and of surrounding normal neurovascular structures. Furthermore, MRI can provide sagittal, coronal and axial images, providing the surgeon with three-dimensional information that is invaluable in preoperative planning. Functional MRI is a relatively new option allowing localization of function. This technique exploits the focal changes in cerebral blood flow that occur in response to stereotypic repetitive activity. The most common application of this technology is the accurate localization of motor, somatosensory or language cortex in relation to tumor. This information can be used to shape surgical strategy, but these findings usually require confirmation by intraoperative recording and stimulation.

Positron emission tomography (PET) is a highly specialized tool for estimating tumor metabolism by measuring tumor uptake of 18-fluoro-2-deoxyglucose or other isotopes. PET scans are used preoperatively to distinguish low-grade from high-grade gliomas, and to identify the most active area of a tumor for biopsy as a means of minimizing sampling error.

Several devices have been developed to improve tumor delineation during surgery, and to identify key functional areas within the surrounding brain. Stereotactic localization by fixed-frame or frameless systems has gained widespread acceptance, and is particularly useful for three-dimensional localization of a tumor and for distinguishing a tumor margin from surrounding brain (Figure 3.1). Intraoperative ultrasound is valuable in localizing subcortical tumors. The optical microscope can identify subtle variations in the colour, texture and vascularity of brain substance, enabling the surgeon to distinguish tumor more easily from surrounding normal brain. Finally, a number of intraoperative functional mapping techniques – such as somatosensory- and motor-evoked potentials, direct stimulation of motor cortex, and electrocorticography – can be used to assist in the resection of lesions bordering eloquent cortex.

Postoperatively, MRI can be used for accurate assessment of the extent of resection, particularly if this is performed within 72 hours of surgery to minimize the confounding effect of surgically induced enhancement produced by reactive inflammation of surrounding tissue.

Stereotactic biopsy is a technique for obtaining diagnostic tissue using a small probe directed by anatomic and geometric guidance at an unseen

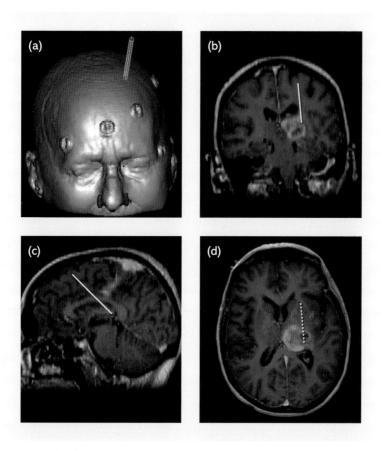

Figure 3.1 (a) Intraoperative computer-assisted three-dimensional reconstruction of a patient with a thalamic glioblastoma. Contrast-enhanced T1-weighted MRI scans demonstrate an enhancing thalamic tumor with central necrosis, and a projected trajectory for frameless stereotactic tumor resection in (b) coronal, (c) sagittal, and (d) axial planes. (Pink squares are midline markers and yellow lines are trajectories.)

target. Several factors are considered before a surgeon chooses stereotactic biopsy over craniotomy for diagnosing a brain lesion (Table 3.1). These include tumor-related factors such as accessibility of the lesion, and patient factors such as serious medical illness or advanced age, which might prohibit radical surgical intervention. Stereotactic biopsy is often considered for tumors situated deep within the cerebrum, the pineal region or posterior fossa.

TABLE 3.1

Factors favoring stereotactic biopsy over resection

Patient factors	Tumor factors
• Elderly	• Deep
• Too ill or too well	• Multiple
• Preference	• Diffuse
	• Small
	• Involving critical areas of brain

The basic technique involves the placement of a stereotactic frame, which is applied to the patient while using a local anaesthetic. Subsequent CT or MRI identifies the coordinates of the target of interest. These coordinates are entered into a computer system, and an appropriate trajectory to the target is generated (Figure 3.2). The patient is taken to the operating theatre, where a burr hole or twist-drill hole is made, and a biopsy needle is inserted into the brain to the designated depth. The needle is rotated and gentle suction applied to obtain the biopsy; the tissue sample is then given to the pathologist for quick-section examination. Postoperatively, the patient is monitored for a few hours, and a postoperative CT is performed to ensure that there is no evidence of hemorrhage.

Stereotactic biopsy is a relatively straightforward neurosurgical procedure. However, there are possible complications, such as intracranial hemorrhage, which occurs in 1.2–7% of patients. Situations associated with increased risk include stereotactic biopsy of highly vascular malignant lesions such as glioblastoma, and eloquent areas of the cerebrum where hemorrhage is more likely to be associated with neurological deficits. If a patient deteriorates significantly as a result of cerebral hemorrhage, immediate craniotomy for hematoma evacuation is mandated.

Stereotactic biopsies are not without shortcomings, the most important of which is a non-diagnostic or misleading result. A stereotactic biopsy samples only a small portion of a lesion, so may

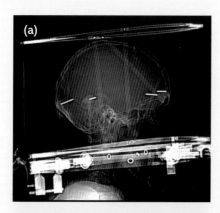

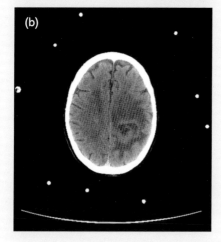

Figure 3.2 (a) Scout radiograph of a patient with a Cosman–Roberts–Wells (CRW) frame for CT-assisted stereotactic biopsy. (b) Image obtained for this patient, showing a deep left parietal glioblastoma.

not be representative of the whole lesion. The overall failure rate for stereotactic biopsies is approximately 8%, with failure appearing to be more common in immunocompromised patients and with lesions that are non-enhancing or non-neoplastic. In the case of gliomas, stereotactic biopsies are associated with approximately 30% imperfect correlation with a fully resected specimen. When the correlation is imperfect, it is usually because the biopsy has underestimated the grade of a tumor. Consequently, a diagnosis based on the histopathology of a stereotactic biopsy must be interpreted with caution. Clinical and imaging features should also be considered, and the diagnosis modified if necessary.

Image-guided surgery describes the use of intraoperative CT and MRI to provide two- and three-dimensional digital information about the normal and pathological anatomy of the brain. This information helps the surgeon to perform a safer and more complete operation. Intraoperative MRI appears to be particularly promising, partly because it circumvents the problems of brain shift and distortion that limit the reliability of CT-based systems.

Surgical navigation systems are increasingly being employed to assist the resection of low- and high-grade gliomas, brain metastases and meningiomas. Use of these navigation systems is also becoming more common in brain biopsy procedures, where they appear to be as reliable as frame-based stereotactic systems for tumor localization and biopsy. Despite the expense of surgical navigation systems, these technologies are becoming an entrenched tool for neurosurgeons, because they promote more efficient, complete and safe tumor resections (Figure 3.3).

Complications following craniotomy for tumor resection are common (occurring in 25–35% of cases), and are listed in Table 3.2.

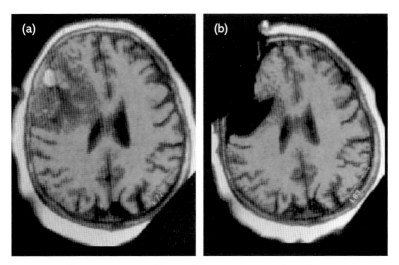

Figure 3.3 Contrast-enhanced T1-weighted axial images of a right frontal glioblastoma (a) before intraoperative MRI-assisted resection; (b) after resection.

TABLE 3.2

Complications of surgery for brain tumors

Neurological

- Worsening of neurological deficit or new neurological deficit

Regional

- Seizure
- Hydrocephalus
- Infection
- Hemorrhage
- Cerebrospinal fluid leak

Systemic

- Deep venous thrombosis/pulmonary embolism
- Infection
- Myocardial infarction
- Fluid/electrolyte disturbance
- Gastrointestinal bleed

Neurological deficit. The most common complication following craniotomy for tumor resection is new or worsening neurological deficit; recent surgical studies report this complication in 10–25% of cases. Risk factors associated with this complication appear to be age greater than 60 years, poor performance status, and a tumor located in an eloquent or deep cerebral location.

Worsening neurological deficits following surgery are due to injury to normal brain, cerebral edema, hematoma, or injury to vascular structures resulting in cerebral ischemia. Postoperative strokes and hematomas are uncommon explanations for such increases in neurological deficit, developing in 1–2% and 1–5%, respectively, of patients having surgery for tumor resection.

Regional complications are classified as CNS events that do not generally result in worsening of the neurological deficit. They occur in 3–5% of all patients undergoing craniotomy for tumor resection, and are more likely to be encountered in elderly patients in poor general health. Common regional complications include postoperative seizures, wound infections, meningitis, hydrocephalus and subgaleal effusions (Figure 3.4).

Seizures in the early postoperative period occur in 0.5–5% of patients after supratentorial craniotomy even with anticonvulsant prophylaxis. Risk factors for postoperative seizures include a history of seizures, surgery adjacent to motor cortex, and postoperative hemorrhage or edema. Although prophylactic anticonvulsants are routinely used in patients undergoing craniotomy for tumor resection, there are no data from randomized trials to support this practice.

Postoperative infections occur in 1–2% of patients undergoing supratentorial craniotomy, and can range from superficial cellulitis to deep infections of bone, surgical cavity and meninges. Most craniotomy infections result from contamination by skin pathogens and the risk can be greatly reduced by use of prophylactic antibiotics.

Systemic complications following craniotomy occur in 5–10% of patients, and commonly include deep venous thrombosis without or with pulmonary embolism, systemic infections, myocardial infarction and electrolyte disturbance. Elderly infirm patients are most susceptible to these morbidities.

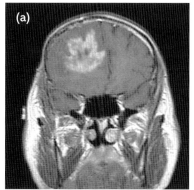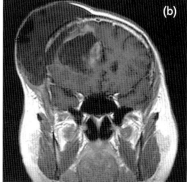

Figure 3.4 (a) T1-weighted magnetic resonance scans with contrast reveal a recurrent right frontal glioma. (b) Following resection, the patient developed a massive subgaleal effusion at the craniotomy site. Decompression was achieved by the insertion of a ventriculoperitoneal shunt.

Mortality associated with craniotomy for resection of intrinsic brain tumors has declined steadily and is presently in the range 1.7–2.7%. Most deaths occur in the elderly with neurological impairment, and are usually due to neurological complications such as intracranial hematoma, edema with cerebral herniation, and early tumor progression.

Radiotherapy

Radiotherapy targets actively dividing cells, with tumor cell death being achieved via induction of DNA damage. The goal of radiotherapy is to achieve maximal tumor control while sparing normal structures from the toxicities of irradiation. The efficacy of radiotherapy depends on the delivery of adequate doses of radiation to the target tissue within the brain. The safety of radiotherapy depends on the relative exclusion of normal brain tissues and other critical structures from exposure to ionising irradiation.

Modern conventional external-beam megavoltage radiotherapy administers irradiation in fractionated doses, thereby allowing normal tissues adequate time to recover from radiation damage. Furthermore, the use of image-guided conformal techniques has enabled radiation oncologists to target the tumor with unprecedented accuracy, so as to minimize the exposure of surrounding normal tissues to ionizing radiation.

Radiotherapy is one of the most effective treatments for brain tumors. It can be curative for some types of brain tumor, such as germinoma, and has a central role in the management of most primary brain tumors, including low-grade and malignant gliomas, where it can reduce the rate of tumor progression and prolong patient survival. Radiotherapy is also the primary palliative modality for the treatment of brain metastases from systemic cancers.

Basic principles. Radiotherapy induces cellular damage by ionizing molecules in DNA, organelles and membranes. The generation of these free radicals can be accentuated by the presence of oxygen, or reversed by naturally occurring free-radical scavengers. The most important cellular target of radiotherapy is DNA, as ionizing irradiation can cause DNA crosslinks and breaks, as well as molecular damage to nucleotides. Although the cell is capable of repairing much of this damage using a variety of 'housekeeping' molecules, when a critical level of damage is reached a process of programmed cell death is triggered via a complicated signal transduction pathway.

Most tumors, including gliomas, cannot be cured by radiotherapy. The radioresistance of tumors depends on several factors, including intrinsic cellular resistance, rapid cell repopulation during radiotherapy and hypoxia, all of which reduce the efficacy of radiotherapy. A number of experimental approaches have been devised to circumvent the radioresistance of tumors. However, the use of hypoxic-cell sensitizers, hyperbaric oxygen, and radiosensitizing molecules such as halogenated pyrimidines has not improved the results of radiotherapy for brain neoplasms.

The toxic effects of radiotherapy on surrounding normal neurovascular structures limits the total dose of radiotherapy that can safely be administered to the target tumor. This obstacle is minimized by delivering radiotherapy in fractions of 1.6–2.0 Gy/day, which reduces the damage sustained by late-responding tissues in the brain. Attempts to improve tumor cell kill rates while preserving normal tissues have included further manipulation of the dose and schedule of radiotherapy. However, these techniques, known as hyperfractionation and accelerated treatment schedules, have failed to improve outcomes for patients with brain neoplasms.

The cells in the brain that are susceptible to the late effects of radiotherapy are vascular endothelial cells and oligodendroglial cells, both of which have prolonged lifespans and low rates of proliferation. Consequently, the late effects of radiotherapy on the brain, namely vascular necrosis and demyelination, are delayed by months to years after cranial irradiation.

Radiotherapeutic techniques. Radiation is usually administered as photons from an external cobalt source or high-energy linear accelerator, but electrons, protons and charged heavy particles have also been used for the treatment of brain tumors. Radiation oncologists aim to deliver the maximal amount of radiation to the tumor while minimizing the dose to the surrounding brain. CT or magnetic resonance scans provide delineation of tumor so that radiation can be delivered accurately to the appropriate target, including a margin of presumed microscopic tumor extension.

For most brain tumors, radiotherapy is considered palliative because it cannot achieve a cure. In some cases, palliative radiotherapy is as short as one or two treatments. Usually, however, it resembles curative radiotherapy schedules, extending over 25–30 treatments in an attempt to achieve protracted tumor control in patients such as those with low-grade gliomas or meningiomas, where a life expectancy of years is anticipated.

External beam radiotherapy is the most common technique for administering irradiation to brain tumors. It employs a number of spatially distributed intersecting beams to deliver radiotherapy to a defined three-dimensional volume. Computer-assisted treatment planning is used to achieve a uniform dose of irradiation to a unique target volume, while delivering a minimum dose to surrounding structures. Treatment is administered in multiple equal doses, usually 25–30 doses for patients with gliomas. To ensure that the same target volume is treated with each dose, patients are immobilized in a fixation mask, and regular imaging of the treatment portals on the linear accelerator ensures accuracy of positioning.

Stereotactic radiotherapy is a precise technique for delivery of external beam radiotherapy. There are two means of administering radiation in this way:

- a multiheaded cobalt unit, known as a gamma knife, which is capable of delivering radiation to a volume of 5–18 mm^3
- a linear accelerator, which is capable of administering radiotherapy in multiple coplanar arcs or multiple coplanar beams.

Single fraction stereotactic radiotherapy is a useful technique for arteriovenous malformations, and has been used for brain metastases. Although it is used for meningiomas, acoustic schwannomas and gliomas, its benefit remains unproven.

It is likely that stereotactic radiotherapy will find application for a broad variety of brain neoplasms, because it enables conventional doses of radiotherapy to be delivered precisely with considerable sparing of surrounding normal structures.

Interstitial radiotherapy involves implantation of radiation sources directly into the tumor. This technique, also known as brachytherapy, permits delivery of very high doses of radiation to the tumor, while exposing the surrounding brain to significantly lower doses. The most common isotopes used in brachytherapy are iodine-125 or iridium-192.

The radiation sources are usually placed in catheters inserted temporarily into the tumor under CT or MRI guidance. Typically, multiple catheters are inserted into a tumor to achieve a homogeneous distribution of radiation (Figure 3.5). An alternative means of local administration involves the placement of radioactive colloid or radiolabeled antibody into a cystic tumor cavity. These novel techniques are highly specialized and remain experimental, with no proven benefit for malignant brain tumors.

Particle-beam therapy. Heavy particles such as protons and neutrons are used in selected centres for specific tumors. These therapies require a cyclotron and are thus not widely available. The main advantage of

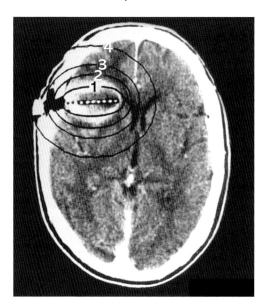

Figure 3.5 Axial CT scan of an iodine-125 implant in a patient with a malignant glioma. Lines 1–4 represent radiation isodoses (e.g. line 1 represents 12 000 cGy, and line 3 represents 2400 cGy).

proton therapy is the ability to circumscribe precisely the target of interest, because protons deposit their energy at the end of their trajectory through tissue. Proton therapy is used for the management of skull base tumors such as chordomas and chondrosarcomas, and pituitary adenomas. Neutron therapy has been of interest in the management of brain tumors because its efficacy is not diminished under hypoxic conditions. Despite these theoretical advantages, there is no evidence that neutron therapy is more effective than other forms of radiotherapy in brain neoplasms.

Complications of cranial radiotherapy. The side effects of radiotherapy to the brain are described chronologically as acute, early delayed and late delayed.

Acute reactions to radiotherapy develop within hours to days of treatment and are transient, manifesting usually as headache or worsening of neurological deficit. These reactions are due to increasing tumor-associated edema and are treated with corticosteroids.

Early delayed toxicities due to cranial irradiation occur 6 weeks to 6 months after completion of radiotherapy, and are presumably the result of reversible demyelination, which causes worsening neurological deficits. This is impossible to distinguish from early tumor progression, but is reversible and can be treated with corticosteroids (Figure 3.6). In addition, many patients experience lethargy, fatigue and mild memory impairment during this time interval, which represent the mild toxicities of radiotherapy.

Late delayed toxicities. The most dreaded complication of radiotherapy to the brain is radionecrosis of white matter (Figure 3.7). This usually develops years after completion of radiotherapy, is indistinguishable clinically and radiographically from tumor progression, and is generally not responsive to corticosteroids. The pathological hallmarks of this condition are demyelination and coagulative necrosis. Another under-reported late effect of cranial radiotherapy is dementia, which ranges clinically from mild cognitive impairment to severe dementia necessitating total care of the affected patient.

A rare late effect of cranial irradiation is neoplasia. Although the precise risk remains undefined, patients receiving brain radiotherapy are

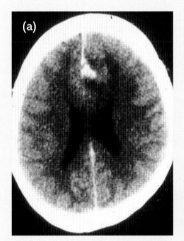
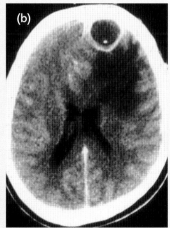

Figure 3.6 (a) Contrast-enhanced CT image of a patient with a left frontal anaplastic astrocytoma before cranial radiotherapy.

(b) The same patient 6 weeks after cranial radiotherapy. The appearance of a new enhancing cystic lesion with increasing edema and mass effect suggests early tumor progression. The patient remained asymptomatic.

(c) Follow-up CT performed 6 months after completion of radiotherapy without further treatment demonstrated regression of the suspicious lesion, suggesting that the radiographic changes causing concern in (b) were due to an early delayed effect of radiotherapy.

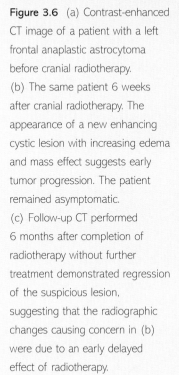
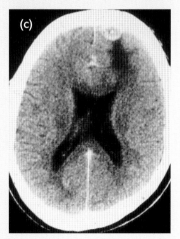

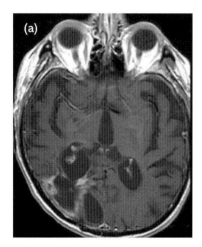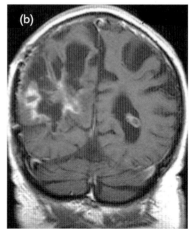

Figure 3.7 Contrast-enhanced MRI of a patient who received brachytherapy for a right parietal anaplastic astrocytoma 12 years earlier. Images demonstrate widespread leukoencephalopathy and cerebral atrophy with stable residual enhancement indicative of cerebral radionecrosis: (a) axial view, (b) coronal view.

at increased risk for the development of meningiomas and gliomas in the treatment field (Figure 3.8). Finally, patients receiving radiotherapy to the parasellar region are at increased risk of visual impairment resulting from damage to the optic pathways, and of hormone deficiency arising from hypothalamic and pituitary dysfunction.

Future radiotherapy trends. Radiotherapy is likely to remain an indispensable treatment modality for brain tumors. Advances will probably be in the realm of novel techniques for delivering increased doses of radiotherapy to the tumor, while limiting toxicity to surrounding normal structures. Image-based three-dimensional conformal techniques for delivering external beam radiotherapy are designed to achieve this goal, and have become standard practice in many centres. However, a full assessment of the benefits of this technique awaits longer-term follow-up.

The value of single fraction radiotherapy administered stereotactically by gamma knife or linear accelerator technologies, compared with conventional fractionated external beam radiotherapy, is unknown and also needs longer-term data to become available.

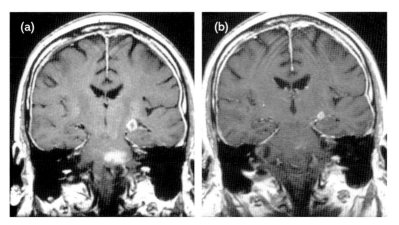

Figure 3.8 Contrast-enhanced coronal MRI of a patient who developed a radiation-induced multifocal glioblastoma multiforme 12 years after receiving radiotherapy for a pituitary adenoma. (a) The glioma developed within the treatment field. (b) Temporary regression was achieved with six cycles of temozolomide chemotherapy.

Chemotherapy

Chemotherapy has a limited but expanding role in the treatment of patients with brain tumors. Many pediatric intracranial tumors are treated primarily with chemotherapy for two reasons. First, tumors common in the pediatric population, such as medulloblastoma and primitive neuroectodermal tumors, are highly chemosensitive. Hence, the addition of chemotherapy to the treatment of these neoplasms has significantly improved outcome and extended survival. Second, the toxic consequences of irradiation on the developing nervous system have stimulated the development of chemotherapy-based strategies that avoid or delay radiotherapy in the pediatric population.

For adults with malignant brain tumors, chemotherapy remains controversial because large randomized clinical trials have failed to show a survival advantage for patients with malignant glioma who received adjuvant chemotherapy. Nevertheless, many patients with malignant gliomas receive chemotherapy at some stage of their illness, because it is a reasonable therapeutic option at recurrence following initial therapy with surgery and irradiation, and because there is a subset of malignant gliomas that are chemosensitive. In particular, malignant oligodendroglial tumors often respond dramatically to chemotherapy, hence this treatment option has become central to the management of these gliomas.

Basic principles. A number of inherent biological issues have hindered the development of effective chemotherapies for primary brain tumors. These issues include the cellular kinetics of brain tumors, inherent or acquired drug resistance, the blood–brain barrier and the potential toxicity of chemotherapy.

Cellular kinetics. Chemotherapeutic agents affect dividing cells. In the normal adult brain, the only cells undergoing division are endothelial cells. For a given tumor, the proportion of cells undergoing division, the rate of this division and the rate of tumor cell death determine tumor growth. Theoretically, the most rapidly growing tumors should be most sensitive to the damaging effects of chemotherapy. Glioblastomas are the most rapidly growing gliomas, with 1–16% of the cells undergoing division at any point in time. Anaplastic and low-grade gliomas have much lower rates of division. Consequently, many chemotherapies have a limited capacity to kill glioma cells, because many are in a quiescent phase of the cell cycle and not susceptible to these agents.

Blood–brain barrier. Endothelial cells with tight junctions and astrocytic foot processes effectively constitute a barrier between the brain parenchyma and circulating blood. Although the blood–brain barrier is altered in high-grade gliomas, there are areas where it remains intact, preventing entry of some chemicals into the tumor.

The ability of a chemotherapeutic agent to penetrate the blood–brain barrier is determined by several factors, including the size of the molecule and its charge, pH, lipid solubility and protein binding. In general, small lipid-soluble molecules with neutral charges are the most effective at crossing this barrier. Other factors influencing penetration of the blood–brain barrier include the degree of tumor vascularity, and blood flow and pressure.

Drug resistance. Malignant gliomas are clonal neoplasms with considerable genetic heterogeneity. Consequently, chemotherapy creates a selective pressure favoring tumor cells that elaborate proteins that are able to circumvent the damaging effects of the chemotherapeutic agents. This development of drug resistance is a common reason for failure of chemotherapy. For example, an enzyme called ^{6}O-methylguanine-DNA-methyltransferase can reverse the damaging effects of nitrosoureas. This enzyme is present in normal cells and brain tumors, and may explain the development of resistance to alkylating agents that is commonly observed in patients with brain tumors.

Toxicity. The use of chemotherapy in patients with brain tumors is limited by the side effects of these compounds. Most agents affect dividing cells, and myelosuppression is common, manifesting most frequently as leukopenia and thrombocytopenia. Moreover, many agents are potentially neurotoxic, which has limited the development of strategies such as intra-arterial chemotherapy that deliver concentrated doses of drug to the brain.

Drug delivery. To be effective, chemotherapy must reach its target. Most drugs for brain tumors are administered orally or intravenously. Agents that are commonly administered by mouth for brain tumors include the alkylating drugs temozolomide and lomustine (CCNU). Concerns with oral delivery include variable absorption from the gut and patient compliance. Most chemotherapeutic agents are delivered intravenously, such as carmustine (BCNU), which is commonly used for malignant glioma. Risks associated with intravenous administration of chemotherapy include local venous complications, cardiac events such as hypotension, and systemic toxicities from the widespread distribution of drug.

As mentioned earlier, the blood–brain barrier presents a challenge to drug delivery in patients with brain tumors. This has resulted in the development of novel delivery techniques, including intra-arterial chemotherapy with or without blood–brain barrier disruption, interstitial chemotherapy with microinfusion pumps, high-dose chemotherapy with stem-cell rescue, and intratumoral polymer placement. All but the last technique are experimental. Recently, carmustine-impregnated biodegradable wafers (Gliadel) applied to the surface of the surgical cavity following tumor resection have been approved for recurrent malignant intracranial glial tumors.

Specific agents. Table 3.3 lists agents commonly used for brain cancer. These drugs have modest activity against brain tumors. Most are administered as single agents, although the combination of procarbazine, lomustine (CCNU) and vincristine (PCV regimen) is commonly used for anaplastic astrocytoma and oligodendroglioma.

Temozolomide is the most recently approved agent for malignant glioma, and is perhaps the most commonly prescribed agent for glioblastoma multiforme and anaplastic astrocytoma (Figure 3.9). In Europe and Canada, it is approved for both diseases at recurrence, but only for recurrent anaplastic astrocytoma in the USA.

It is an oral agent and works by alkylating DNA at multiple locations, most commonly guanine. The formation of DNA crosslinks produces single- and double-stranded breaks, ultimately resulting in tumor cell death. Temozolomide also depletes O6-methylguanine-DNA-methyltransferase, the enzyme responsible for DNA repair and resistance against agents such as temozolomide. Toxicities are generally mild and include nausea, vomiting and non-cumulative myelosuppression.

TABLE 3.3

Chemotherapeutic agents commonly used for brain tumors

- Nitrosoureas
  - Carmustine (BCNU)
  - Lomustine (CCNU)
- Procarbazine
- Platinum analogs
  - Carboplatin
  - Cisplatin
- Etoposide
- Temozolomide
- PCV regimen (procarbazine, lomustine (CCNU), vincristine)
- Cytarabine (ara-C)
- Methotrexate

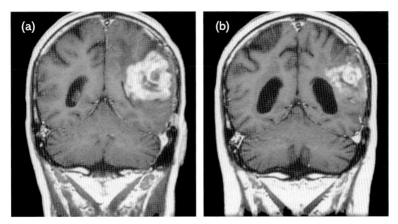

Figure 3.9 (a) Contrast-enhanced coronal MRI of a 55-year-old man with an enlarging parieto-occipital glioblastoma 6 months after completion of cranial radiotherapy. (b) Significant tumor regression was noted after one cycle of temozolomide chemotherapy.

Nitrosoureas have been the most widely used group of drugs for patients with brain tumors. The most commonly prescribed agents in this group are lomustine (CCNU) and carmustine (BCNU), given orally and intravenously, respectively. Nitrosoureas exert their antiproliferative effects by DNA alkylation. Toxicities include nausea and vomiting, cumulative and prolonged myelosuppression, and pulmonary fibrosis after extended exposure. These agents are active against glioblastoma multiforme, anaplastic astrocytoma and oligodendroglioma, medulloblastoma and primitive neuroectodermal tumors (PNETs), and various low-grade gliomas.

Procarbazine is a cell-cycle non-specific alkylating agent administered orally. It inhibits DNA, RNA and protein synthesis. Its major toxicities include rash, nausea and vomiting, and myelosuppression. It is also a weak inhibitor of monoamine oxidase, and can cause vascular and neurological side effects if given with drugs and food that contain tyramine. It is active against a variety of brain neoplasms, including high-grade gliomas, medulloblastomas and PNETs, and lymphoma.

Vincristine, a vinca alkaloid, inhibits microtubulin formation by depolymerization, causing cell cycle arrest at mitosis. It is administered

43

Key points – treatment

- Magnetic resonance imaging can suggest a diagnosis of a brain tumor, but surgery is always necessary to provide tissue for pathological diagnosis (except in the case of diffuse pontine glioma).
- Stereotactic biopsy is a safe procedure for obtaining diagnostic tissue, but sampling error may result in the tumor grade being underestimated.
- Image-guided surgery facilitates radical resection of intracranial tumors.
- Elderly patients with poor neurological function are at highest risk of morbidity and mortality following craniotomy for tumor resection.
- Following surgery, radiotherapy is the most effective treatment for long-term control of most intracranial neoplasms.
- Radiotherapy is associated with considerable brain side effects, including late toxicities such as dementia and cerebral radionecrosis.
- Conformal radiotherapy, stereotactic radiosurgery and radiotherapy are emerging techniques designed to provide maximal radiation dose to the tumor while sparing normal tissues.
- Inherent or acquired drug resistance and the blood–brain barrier are important factors limiting the efficacy of chemotherapy in patients with brain tumors.

intravenously and is widely used for the treatment of brain tumors, most commonly as part of the PCV chemotherapy regimen. Toxicity is primarily neurological, and can be dose-limiting. Common side effects are peripheral sensorimotor or autonomic neuropathies. Vincristine is active against high- and low-grade glial neoplasms, medulloblastomas and PNETs, and lymphoma.

Platinum analogs. Cisplatin and carboplatin cause DNA damage by intrastrand and interstrand crosslinking. These agents can be administered intra-arterially, but are more commonly given intravenously. Major toxicities are neuropathy, sensorineural hearing loss and nephropathy for cisplatin, and myelosuppression, nausea and emesis for carboplatin. These analogs have demonstrated single-agent activity against a spectrum of primary brain tumors, including malignant gliomas, medulloblastoma and PNETs, ependymomas and germ cell tumors.

New agents. A greater role for chemotherapy in the management of primary brain tumors awaits the development of better anticancer drugs. Novel therapies that target growth factor signaling pathways, angiogenesis and tumor invasion are presently undergoing clinical investigation in patients with brain tumors. Table 3.4 lists selected new agents that are being investigated for glioma and indicates their cellular targets. It is hoped that these novel theoretical strategies for combating cancer will have demonstrable efficacy and soon become part of standard therapy for patients with malignant brain tumors.

TABLE 3.4

New therapeutic agents for gliomas

Agent	Mechanism of action
Imatinib (Gleevec, Glivec)	Platelet derived growth factor receptor tyrosine kinase inhibitor
Gefitinib (Iressa)	Epidermal growth factor receptor tyrosine kinase inhibitor
Erlotinib (Tarceva)	Epidermal growth factor receptor tyrosine kinase inhibitor
Tamoxifen	Protein kinase C inhibitor
Thalidomide	Tumor angiogenesis inhibitor
Retinoids	Differentiating agent
Phenylacetate	Differentiating agent
PTK787	Tumor angiogenesis inhibitor

Key references

Apuzzo MLJ, Chandrasoma PT, Cohen D et al. Computed imaging stereotaxy: experience and perspective related to 500 procedures applied to brain masses. *Neurosurgery* 1987;20:930–7.

Apuzzo MLJ. New dimensions of neurosurgery in the realm of high technology: possibilities, practicalities, realities. *Neurosurgery* 1996;38:625–39.

Berger MS, Ojemann GA, Lettich E. Neurophysiological monitoring to facilitate resection during astrocytoma surgery. *Neurosurg Clin N Am* 1990;1:65–80.

Bernstein M, Parrent AG. Complications of CT-guided stereotactic biopsy of intra-axial brain lesions. *J Neurosurg* 1994;81: 165–8.

Chandler KL, Prados MD. Chemotherapy of brain tumors: clinical aspects. In: Morantz RA, Walsh JW, eds. *Brain Tumors, a Comprehensive Text.* New York: Marcel Dekker, 1994:731–44.

Fadul C, Wood J, Thaler H et al. Morbidity and mortality of craniotomy for excision of supratentorial gliomas. *Neurology* 1988;38:1374–9.

Fine HA, Dear JGB, Loeffler JS et al. Meta-analysis of radiation therapy with and without adjuvant chemotherapy for malignant gliomas in adults. *Cancer* 1993;71:2585–97.

Grieg NH. Optimizing drug delivery to brain tumors. *Cancer Treat Rev* 1987;14:1–28.

Gutin PH, Leibel SA, Sheline GA. *Radiation Injury to the Nervous System.* New York: Raven Press, 1991.

Hamilton RJ, Sweeney PJ, Pelizzari CA et al. Functional imaging in treatment planning of brain lesions. *Int J Radiat Oncol Biol Phys* 1997;37:181–8.

Hammoud MA, Ligon R, Elsouki R et al. Use of intraoperative ultrasound for localizing tumors and determining the extent of resection: a comparative study with magnetic resonance imaging. *J Neurosurg* 1996;84:737–41.

Kelly PJ, Kall BA, Goerss S, Earnest F. Computer-assisted stereotaxic laser resection of intra-axial brain neoplasms. *J Neurosurg* 1986;64: 427–39.

Laperriere NJ, Leung PM, McKenzie S et al. Randomized study of brachytherapy in the initial management of patients with malignant astrocytoma. *Int J Radiat Oncol Biol Phys* 1998;41:1005–11.

Leibel SA, Scott CB, Loeffler JS. Contemporary approaches to the treatment of malignant gliomas with radiation therapy. *Semin Oncol* 1994;21:198–219.

Levin VA. Pharmacokinetics and central nervous system chemotherapy. In: Hellmann K, Carter SK, eds. *Fundamentals of Cancer Chemotherapy*. New York: McGraw-Hill, 1986:28–40.

Loeffler JS, Shrieve DC, Wen PY et al. Radiosurgery for intracranial malignancies. In: Purdy JA. Advances in three-dimensional treatment planning and conformal dose delivery. *Semin Oncol* 1997; 26:655–72

Schwade J, ed. *Seminars in Radiation Oncology*. Vol 5. Philadelphia: WB Saunders, 1995:225–34.

Raju MR. Proton radiobiology, radiosurgery and radiotherapy. *Int J Radiat Oncol Biol Phys* 1995;67:237–59.

Ron E, Modan B, Boice JD et al. Tumors of the brain and nervous system after radiotherapy in childhood. *N Engl J Med* 1988;319: 1033–9.

Sawaya R, Hammoud M, Schoppa D et al. Neurosurgical outcomes in a modern series of 400 craniotomies for treatment of parenchymal tumors. *Neurosurgery* 1998;42: 1044–56

Yung WKA. Temozolomide in malignant glioma. *Seminars Oncol* 2000;27:27–34.

Improvements in therapy for systemic cancer has resulted in an increase in the number of patients living long enough to develop symptomatic brain metastasis. Indeed, brain metastases are the most common intracranial tumor. Therefore, new strategies to prevent and treat brain metastases will become increasingly important.

Currently, 1 in 4 patients with cancer will develop a brain metastasis; patients with melanoma, lung or breast cancer are at the greatest risk (Table 4.1). Most patients present with headaches or focal neurological deficits; 20% or more present with or develop seizures. Radiographically, metastases are ring enhancing lesions, most often located at the gray–white matter junction. There is often significant surrounding edema. About half are single lesions (Figure 4.1); the remainder are multiple (Figures 4.2 and 4.3). Skull and dural metastases are most commonly seen in association with prostate and breast cancer.

Patients with a new diagnosis of brain metastasis should be systemically restaged as appropriate for their primary tumor. A treatment algorithm for newly diagnosed brain metastasis is shown in Figure 4.4.

TABLE 4.1

Risk of brain metastasis by tumor type

Small-cell lung cancer	Up to 80%
Non-small-cell lung cancer	25–30%
Melanoma	Up to 50% (50–75% autopsy)
Renal	5–10%
Breast	10–20%
Testicular	8–15%
Choriocarcinoma	10–15%

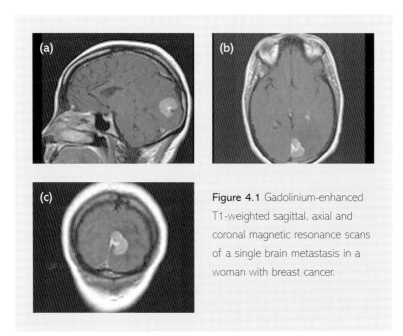

Figure 4.1 Gadolinium-enhanced T1-weighted sagittal, axial and coronal magnetic resonance scans of a single brain metastasis in a woman with breast cancer.

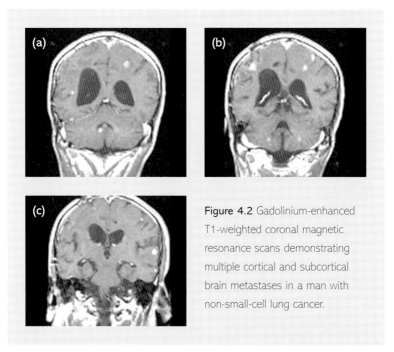

Figure 4.2 Gadolinium-enhanced T1-weighted coronal magnetic resonance scans demonstrating multiple cortical and subcortical brain metastases in a man with non-small-cell lung cancer.

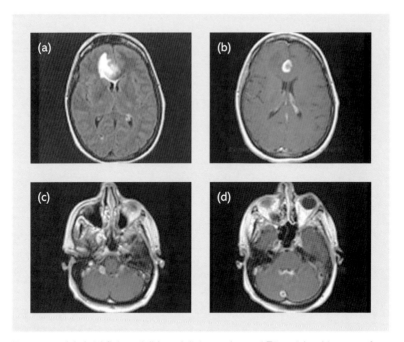

Figure 4.3 (a) Axial flair and (b) gadolinium-enhanced T1-weighted images of a frontal metastasis with significant surrounding edema. (c) and (d) demonstrate additional superficial metastases and leptomeningeal dissemination.

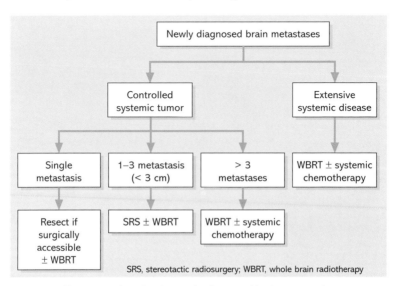

Figure 4.4 Treatment algorithm for newly diagnosed brain metastasis.

Symptomatic management

Symptomatic management can result in a significant improvement in quality of life for patients with brain metastases. Vigilance for less common complications of brain metastases, such as the syndrome of inappropriate antidiuretic hormone secretion (SIADH), is critical.

Vasogenic edema secondary to metastases typically responds to treatment with corticosteroids within a matter of hours. Dexamethasone is the corticosteroid most often used. For initial symptom control, it can be administered in two, three or four daily doses, with each dose between 16 mg and 100 mg. Unfortunately, there are significant side effects associated with corticosteroids, including but not limited to myopathy, hyperglycemia, edema, weight gain, avascular necrosis and psychosis. All patients on prolonged corticosteroids should receive prophylactic therapy for *Pneumocystis carinii* pneumonia. Steroids should be tapered as rapidly as possible (decreasing the dose every 3 days, as tolerated) to minimize side effects. Eliminating doses given late in the day and minimizing multiple daily doses may help to limit the side effects.

Anticonvulsants are indicated for any patient presenting with a seizure. Prophylactic anticonvulsants have not been shown to be effective and therefore only complicate patient management, increasing the risk of medication-related side effects. Non-convulsive status epilepticus should be considered in any patient with an altered level of consciousness.

Radiotherapy and surgery

Standard therapy for a patient with newly diagnosed brain metastasis is whole-brain radiotherapy. A total dose of 3 000 cGy is administered in 10 daily doses of 300 cGy. Prognosis following standard therapy is poor, with average survival in the range 3–4 months. About 50% of patients die from progressive neurological disease; the remainder die as a result of systemic tumor progression.

Aggressive focused management of brain metastases may improve the prognosis for some patients. Those with a single brain metastasis located in a surgically accessible region clearly benefit from a combination of surgical resection and whole-brain radiotherapy. Similar results have been reported with the use of stereotactic radiosurgery. Median survival with either of these approaches is 8–9 months in this group of patients.

Controversy still surrounds several specific issues. First, there is no consensus on the number and size of lesions that are appropriate to treat with stereotactic radiosurgery. Second, the optimal timing of whole-brain radiotherapy following surgical resection or stereotactic radiosurgery therapy is unclear. There are data that suggest early whole-brain radiotherapy improves neurological control, but there is no clear survival benefit. As a result, many practitioners are inclined to defer whole-brain radiotherapy until there is progressive disease in the brain. This strategy may minimize treatment-related neurocognitive deficits and permit much needed palliation at a future time-point. These results, while encouraging, have been obtained in highly selected patient populations, most of whom had a high Karnofsky performance status, limited systemic tumor burden and small brain metastases; such patients have an inherently better prognosis. The results may therefore not be easily extrapolated to all patients.

Recent work published by the Radiation Therapy Oncology Group (RTOG) has delineated specific prognostic categories for patients with newly diagnosed brain metastases (Table 4.2). This may be helpful in determining appropriate treatment options and long-term plans (e.g. hospice care) for individual patients. Application of these categories to future studies will allow treatment results to be generalized to larger groups of patients.

Chemotherapy

Use of chemotherapy in the treatment of brain metastases has generally proved disappointing. Unfortunately, by the time most patients develop brain metastases, they have already been exposed to the most effective chemotherapeutic agents and the metastatic clones are relatively chemoresistant. Although the blood–brain barrier is disrupted in patients with brain metastases, water-soluble chemotherapy may not penetrate sufficiently to attain a therapeutic concentration.

In spite of this, chemotherapy may be useful in treating some individuals with brain metastases. Newly diagnosed patients who are

TABLE 4.2

Radiation Therapy Oncology Group recursive partitioning analysis classification

Class	Age (years)	KPS	Systemic extent of disease	Survival (months)	Recommended treatment
I*	≤ 65	≥70	Controlled primary tumor; no other systemic metastases	7.1	Aggressive focused therapy if possible ± whole-brain radiotherapy
II	Not specified	≥ 70	Not specified	4.2	Whole-brain radiotherapy; consider aggressive focused therapy in patients with controlled systemic tumor and ≤ three brain metastases
III	Not specified	< 70	Not specified	2.3	Whole-brain radiotherapy or palliative care; more aggressive therapy should be considered only in highly selected patients

*Class I comprises fewer than 20% of all patients
KPS, Karnofsky performance status (a KPS of 70 or better implies that the patient is able to care for himself or herself

chemotherapy naïve and neurologically asymptomatic may respond favorably to systemic chemotherapy. They should be followed closely with serial MRI and neurological examinations to monitor their response to treatment. In particular, patients with brain metastases from small-cell lung cancer, breast cancer, testicular cancer or choriocarcinoma may have a better than average response to chemotherapy.

Chemotherapy may also be combined with whole-brain radiotherapy in an attempt to improve the outcome compared with either modality alone. A study by the European Organization for Research on Treatment of Cancer (EORTC) found a significant survival advantage for small-cell lung cancer patients treated with teniposide in combination with whole-brain radiotherapy, when compared with teniposide alone. Similarly, Antonadou et al. found a significant improvement in radiographic response for patients with newly diagnosed brain metastases who were treated with temozolomide in combination with whole-brain radiotherapy, when compared with whole-brain radiotherapy alone.

Finally, chemotherapy may be useful in the setting of recurrent brain metastases. At recurrence, most patients have multiple lesions that are not amenable to radiosurgery or focal therapy. Furthermore, the majority have active and often symptomatic systemic tumor. This clinical scenario makes palliative chemotherapy an appropriate intervention. We recently completed a trial of single-agent temozolomide therapy for patients with recurrent brain metastases and found that median survival was improved when compared with historical controls.

Key points – brain metastases

- Improvements in therapy for systemic cancer have resulted in an increase in the number of patients living long enough to develop symptomatic brain metastasis. It is likely that this trend will continue. Therefore, new strategies to prevent and treat brain metastases will become increasingly important.
- Patients with a new diagnosis of brain metastasis should be systemically restaged as appropriate for their primary tumor.
- Although the average prognosis for an individual with brain metastasis is poor, selected patients will benefit significantly from aggressive local therapy or judicious use of chemotherapy.

Key references

Abrey LE, Olson JD, Raizer JJ et al. A phase II trial of temozolomide for patients with recurrent or progressive brain metastases. *J Neurooncol* 2001;53:259–65.

Antonadou D, Paraskevaidis M, Sarris G et al. Phase II randomized trial of temozolomide and concurrent radiotherapy in patients with brain metastases. *J Clin Oncol* 2002; 20:3644–50.

Gaspar LE, Scott C, Murray K, Curran W. Validation of the RTOG recursive partitioning analysis (RPA) classification for brain metastases. *Int J Radiat Oncol Biol Phys* 2000; 47:1001–6.

Patchell RA, Tibbs PA, Walsh JW et al. A randomized trial of surgery in the treatment of single metastases to the brain. *N Engl J Med* 1990; 322:494–500.

Postmus PE, Haaxma-Reiche H, Smit EF et al. Treatment of brain metastases of small-cell lung cancer: comparing teniposide and teniposide with whole-brain radiotherapy – a phase III study of the European Organization for the Research and Treatment of Cancer Lung Cancer Cooperative Group. *J Clin Oncol* 2000;18:3400–8.

Sneed PK, Suh JH, Goetsch SJ et al. A multi-institutional review of radiosurgery alone vs radiosurgery with whole brain radiotherapy as the initial management of brain metastases. *Int J Radiat Oncol Biol Phys* 2002;53:519–26.

Gliomas are primary brain tumors that are derived from three basic types of glial cells: astrocytes, ependymal cells and oligodendrocytes. Together, astrocytomas, oligodendrogliomas and ependymomas account for 67.6% of all primary brain tumors. The different types of gliomas share a number of characteristics, including indistinct margins that make complete surgical resection impossible, incurability, genetic instability and increasing malignancy over time, as well as a tendency for local recurrence following initial treatment. Common presenting symptoms include seizures, focal neurological deficits and headache.

Several systems exist for the pathological diagnosis of gliomas, the most frequently used of which is the WHO classification (Table 5.1). Astrocytic gliomas are the most common type, and include anaplastic astrocytomas and the highly malignant glioblastoma multiforme that can arise de novo or from a pre-existing low-grade astrocytoma. All gliomas have the potential to become malignant neoplasms through a process of malignant degeneration caused by a series of genetic aberrations that are currently being defined (Table 5.2). The prognosis for patients with malignant gliomas is influenced most by histological grade and age.

Glioblastoma multiforme

Glioblastoma multiforme is the most common and aggressive of all gliomas. This category of tumor accounts for 45–50% of all gliomas, arising most frequently in individuals aged 45–65 years. The male to female ratio is approximately 1.5:1. Glioblastomas usually arise in the deep white matter of the cerebrum, with the temporal and frontal lobes being the most common sites.

A diagnosis of glioblastoma multiforme can be suspected on the basis of imaging studies, where the tumor appears as a heterogeneous enhancing mass with or without a necrotic or cystic core. The margins are usually indistinct, and surrounding edema is usually prominent (Figure 5.1). MRI is more accurate than CT for determining tumor size

TABLE 5.1

Modified World Health Organization classification of gliomas

Astrocytomas

- Glioblastoma multiforme
- Anaplastic astrocytoma
- Astrocytoma
- Pilocytic astrocytoma

Oligodendrogliomas

- Anaplastic oligodendroglioma
- Oligodendroglioma

Mixed gliomas

- Anaplastic oligoastrocytomas
- Oligoastrocytoma

Ependymomas

- Anaplastic ependymomas
- Ependymoma
- Myxopapillary ependymoma

TABLE 5.2

Key genetic events in the development of gliomas

Low-grade astrocytoma

- p53 mutation
- PDGF-A, PDGFR-α amplification

Anaplastic astrocytoma

- LOH 19q
- RB alteration

Glioblastoma multiforme

- EGFR amplification and overexpression
- p16 deletion
- LOH 10
- RB alteration

Oligodendroglioma and anaplastic oligodendroglioma

- LOH 1p and 19q

PDGF-A, platelet-derived growth factor, subunit A; PDGFR-α platelet-derived growth factor receptor α subunit; LOH, loss of heterozygosity; RB, retinoblastoma gene; EGFR, epidermal growth factor receptor

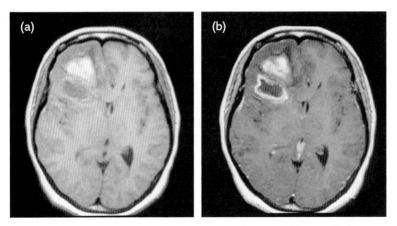

Figure 5.1 (a) Axial MRI of a patient with a right frontal glioblastoma before contrast administration, showing a lesion with cystic necrosis and intratumoral hemorrhage, and surrounding edema and mass effect. (b) Following administration of contrast, the margin of the tumor enhances uniformly.

and extent. As with all brain tumors, pathology is required for a definitive diagnosis. The histological hallmarks of glioblastomas include cellular and nuclear pleomorphism, hypervascularity, brisk mitoses and, usually, necrosis (Figure 5.2).

Like all gliomas, glioblastomas are infiltrative tumors. Hence, the morbidity and poor prognosis associated with these tumors is the result of invasion of the surrounding brain. Glioblastomas are highly aggressive and survival statistics remain poor. Median survival for patients offered only supportive care is approximately 14 weeks. However, aggressive treatment that includes maximal surgical resection followed by radiotherapy has extended median survival to approximately 9–12 months.

Several prognostic factors have been identified for glioblastomas, with more favorable outcomes being associated with younger age, greater preoperative and postoperative performance score, maximal surgical resection, and the absence of necrosis.

The role of adjuvant chemotherapy remains controversial. No randomized phase III study has demonstrated improved survival for patients receiving chemotherapy as part of their initial treatment. Nevertheless, most individuals with glioblastomas will receive

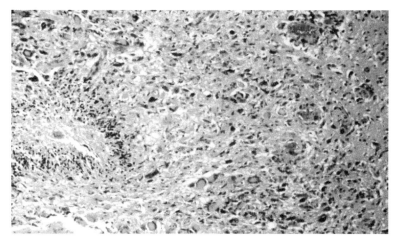

Figure 5.2 Photomicrograph of a glioblastoma specimen stained with hematoxylin and eosin demonstrates hypercellularity with frequent mitoses, considerable cellular and nuclear pleomorphism, hypervascularity, the formation of pseudopallisades and tumor necrosis – all hallmark features of glioblastoma multiforme.

chemotherapy at some stage of their illness, because there is tumor recurrence within two years of the initial diagnosis in the vast majority of patients. Tumor recurrence is usually local and confined to the brain. At recurrence, further surgery and chemotherapy can extend life in a minority of patients.

The most common chemotherapeutic agents in current use for malignant gliomas are listed in Table 5.3. A number of experimental treatments are under investigation for glioblastoma, including immunotherapy, viral therapy, signal transduction inhibitors and anti-angiogenic agents.

Anaplastic astrocytoma

Between 10% and 30% of all gliomas are anaplastic astrocytomas. These tumors tend to arise in individuals who are aged 35–55 years. Males are slightly over-represented, with the male to female ratio being 1.2:1. Anaplastic astrocytomas typically appear as solid masses with surrounding edema and mass effect on MRI scans. Contrast enhancement is variable, although present in 80–90% of cases.

TABLE 5.3

Antineoplastic agents commonly used for gliomas

- Nitrosoureas
  - Carmustine (BCNU)
  - Lomustine (CCNU)
- Procarbazine
- Platinum analogs
  - Carboplatin
  - Cisplatin
- Etoposide
- Temozolomide
- PCV regimen (procarbazine, lomustine and vincristine)

Anaplastic astrocytomas are associated with better survival statistics than glioblastomas, with a median survival of 24–36 months with treatment. Aggressive treatment including maximal surgery and radiotherapy with or without adjuvant chemotherapy has resulted in reported median survival in excess of 5 years in some series. The use of adjuvant chemotherapy is more common in patients with anaplastic astrocytomas than in those with glioblastomas, but remains controversial. The most frequently used agents include temozolomide and the combination of procarbazine, lomustine (CCNU) and vincristine (PCV chemotherapy).

Despite initial attempts at control, recurrence is expected, usually as a glioblastoma. At recurrence, the treatment options include further surgery, chemotherapy or experimental agents.

Low-grade astrocytoma

Low-grade astrocytomas account for 5–10% of all gliomas and typically arise in individuals aged 30–50 years. Most patients present with seizures only and have no fixed neurological deficits. The median survival for adults receiving treatment for low-grade astrocytic gliomas is in the range 4–7 years, although some series report survival rates in excess of 10 years.

The diagnosis of a low-grade astrocytic glioma can almost be established by its unique imaging features. Typically, MRI reveals a non-enhancing hypointense lesion on T1-weighted images after contrast administration, and a sharply demarcated hyperintense lesion with minimal or no surrounding edema on T2-weighted images (Figure 5.3). Patients who present with seizures only and have typical radiographic features of a low-grade astrocytic glioma are often observed for a period of time using serial imaging before any surgical intervention is undertaken. Nevertheless, tissue is required for a firm diagnosis. This is preferably obtained during maximal surgical resection, or using stereotactic or open biopsy for inaccessible lesions.

Following surgery, radiotherapy is often administered, although the timing and dose of irradiation remain under debate. Several large randomized trials designed to address the controversies regarding radiotherapy have recently been reported. The current recommendation for low-grade astrocytic gliomas is deferred radiotherapy, given at lower doses (typically 50–54 Gy). Deferred radiotherapy refers to withholding irradiation until there is evidence of radiographic or clinical progression.

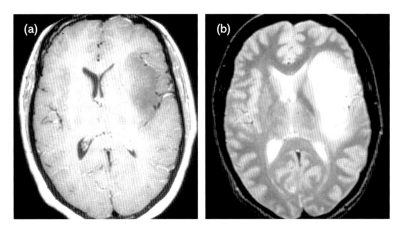

Figure 5.3 (a) Contrast-enhanced axial MRI of a patient with a low-grade astrocytoma of the left insular region. The tumor is uniformly hypointense without contrast enhancement. (b) The T2-weighted image provides better demarcation of a uniformly hyperintense lesion, and is highly suggestive of the underlying pathological diagnosis.

Several prognostic factors for early recurrence have been identified. These factors include age greater than 40 years, fixed neurological deficits, and tumor enhancement or mass effect on imaging. Patients who have one or more of these poor prognostic factors are often treated early with surgery, followed by postoperative irradiation.

Chemotherapy has no established role in the initial management of low-grade astrocytomas. However, these tumors have the potential for dedifferentiation to a more malignant phenotype. Hence, at recurrence these neoplasms are often frankly malignant, and chemotherapy is commonly administered at this time with modest results but poor survival statistics.

Anaplastic oligodendroglioma and oligodendroglioma

Oligodendroglial tumors presumably arise from oligodendrocytes or their precursors, and account for 5–25% of primary brain tumors. Oligodendrogliomas can be a challenging diagnosis for a pathologist, largely because there is no immunohistochemical marker specific for oligodendrocytes. According to the WHO classification system, three types of oligodendrogliomas can be distinguished: low-grade oligodendroglioma, mixed glioma with features of both astrocytoma and oligodendroglioma, and malignant oligodendroglioma.

The epidemiology of oligodendrogliomas and anaplastic oligodendrogliomas is similar to their astrocytic counterparts. However, oligodendroglial tumors are generally associated with a better prognosis than astrocytic neoplasms. Median survival estimates for low-grade and anaplastic oligodendrogliomas have been reported to be approximately 15 years and 4 years, respectively. This may in part be due to the remarkable sensitivity of oligodendroglial tumors to radiotherapy and chemotherapy (Figure 5.4).

Anaplastic oligodendrogliomas have been reported to be particularly chemosensitive, with documented responses to numerous agents including nitrosoureas, temozolomide, procarbazine and the combination chemotherapy PCV. Recently, a subset of anaplastic oligodendrogliomas that have loss of heterozygosity of chromosome 1p and 19q have been shown to be predictably chemosensitive.

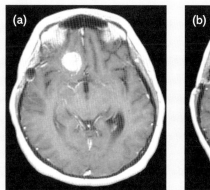 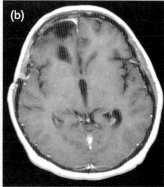

Figure 5.4 (a) Contrast-enhanced axial MRI of a patient with a right frontal anaplastic oligodendroglioma before four cycles of chemotherapy with procarbazine, lomustine and vincristine. (b) Same patient, showing a complete radiographic response to treatment.

Currently, chemotherapy is routinely administered as part of initial treatment for patients with anaplastic oligodendrogliomas. Surgery is also important as a part of initial treatment and for diagnosis.

Results of a recently completed phase III trial, in which patients with newly diagnosed anaplastic oligodendrogliomas were randomized to postoperative radiotherapy with or without PCV chemotherapy, are awaited with interest. When they become available, these results should determine the role of adjuvant chemotherapy for this disease, including the optimum timing for administering such agents.

Low-grade oligodendrogliomas are also sensitive to chemo-therapeutic agents, although the role of chemotherapy in patients with this tumor type is less established. Conventional postoperative treatment for low-grade oligodendrogliomas is similar to treatment for low-grade astrocytomas, namely radiotherapy.

Pilocytic astrocytoma

Pilocytic astrocytomas account for fewer than 5% of gliomas. They are characteristically pediatric brain tumors, although 25% occur in individuals over the age of 18 years. Signs and symptoms are related to tumor location, and are usually insidious because these tumors are indolent. Most commonly, pilocytic astrocytomas arise in the cerebellum, optic pathways, diencephalon and brainstem (Figure 5.5).

Diagnosis is established pathologically. These tumors have characteristic features including well-differentiated astrocytes, Rosenthal fibers, bundles of neurofibrils and microcysts. Nuclear atypia and mitoses do not denote malignancy, although rare pilocytic astrocytomas exhibit clinically malignant behavior.

Pilocytic astrocytomas usually have a well-defined border, which makes surgical resection the preferred treatment whenever possible. Complete surgical resection of pilocytic astrocytomas can be curative, and has been associated with 95% disease-free survival at 25 years for patients with cerebellar tumors. For patients with supratentorial pilocytic astrocytomas, 10-year survival rates of 80–100% have been reported following surgery. The management of pilocytic astrocytomas of the optic pathways remains controversial, but most resectable lesions are excised, particularly if vision is threatened.

Recurrence of pilocytic astrocytomas is managed by reoperation if possible, or by radiotherapy. For very young patients who should not receive irradiation, chemotherapy has been administered with reasonable response rates but poor survival.

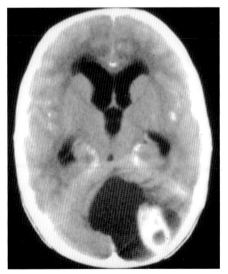

Figure 5.5 Contrast-enhanced CT scan of a 7-year-old boy with a cerebellar astrocytoma that had resulted in obstructive hydrocephalus. The imaging features of a large cystic mass and an intensely enhancing mural nodule without enhancement of the cyst wall are typical for this neoplasm.

> **Key points – gliomas**
>
> - The prognosis for patients with malignant gliomas is influenced most by histological grade and age.
> - Glioblastoma multiforme is the most common and aggressive of all gliomas.
> - Surgery is the principal initial treatment for gliomas. The benefit of extensive surgery versus limited resection or biopsy is controversial.
> - Postoperative radiotherapy delays tumor progression and prolongs life for patients with malignant glioma.
> - Adjuvant chemotherapy for malignant gliomas is controversial. Chemotherapy administered for tumor recurrence or progression is palliative.
> - Anaplastic oligodendroglioma is a chemosensitive tumor. The appropriate timing of chemotherapy is controversial.
> - Observation may be an appropriate initial strategy for patients with low-grade gliomas. The timing and extent of surgery for low-grade glioma is controversial, as is the timing and dose of radiotherapy.

Ependymoma

Ependymomas are uncommon but clinically important gliomas that account for approximately 2–9% of all brain neoplasms. They are most prevalent in patients aged 5–15 years, and represent the third most common intracranial neoplasm in childhood. Ependymomas can arise anywhere in the neuraxis, but are most frequently found in the posterior fossa.

The behavior of ependymomas is unpredictable; both pathologically anaplastic and non-anaplastic ependymomas can behave in a malignant fashion. The primary therapy for these tumors is surgical, and a complete resection can be curative. For malignant tumors, or recurrent ependymomas following surgical resection, radiotherapy is often indicated.

65

The role of chemotherapy in this disease is poorly defined. Response to single agents such as lomustine, etoposide and platinum analogs has been documented, but adjuvant chemotherapy is administered only to younger patients as a means of avoiding cranial irradiation. More commonly, chemotherapy is given for progressive or recurrent disease following surgical and radiotherapeutic failure, and has only modest impact.

Key references

Cairncross JG, Macdonald DR. Successful chemotherapy for recurrent malignant oligodendroglioma. *Ann Neurol* 1988;23:360–4.

Cairncross G, Macdonald D, Ludwin S et al. Chemotherapy for anaplastic oligodendroglioma. *J Clin Oncol* 1994;12:2013–21.

Cairncross JG, Ueki K, Zlatescu MC et al. Specific genetic predictors of chemotherapeutic response and survival in patients with anaplastic oligodendrogliomas. *J Natl Cancer Inst* 1998;90:1473–9.

Chang CH, Horton J, Schoenfeld D et al. Comparison of postoperative radiotherapy and combined postoperative radiotherapy and chemotherapy in the multidisciplinary management of malignant gliomas. *Cancer* 1983;52:997–1007.

Fine HF. The basis for current recommendations for malignant gliomas. *J Neurooncol* 1994;20:111–20.

Karim A, Maat B, Hatlevoli R et al. A randomized trial on dose–response in radiation therapy of low-grade cerebral glioma: European Organization for Research and Treatment of Cancer (EORTC) study 22844. *Int J Radiat Oncol Biol Phys* 1996;36:549—56.

Karim ABMF, Afra D, Cornu P et al. Randomized trial on the efficacy of radiotherapy for cerebral low-grade glioma in the adult: European Organization for Research and Treatment of Cancer study 22845 with the Medical Research Council study BR04: an interim analysis. *Int J Radiat Oncol Biol Phys* 2002;52:316–24.

Levin V, Silver P, Hannigan J et al. Superiority of post-radiotherapy adjuvant chemotherapy with CCNU, procarbazine and vincristine (PCV) over BCNU for anaplastic gliomas: NCOG 6G61 final report. *Int J Radiat Oncol Biol Phys* 1990;18:321–4.

Mason WP, Krol GS, DeAngelis LM. Low-grade oligodendroglioma responds to chemotherapy. *Neurology* 1996;46:203–7.

Mork SJ, Loken AC. Ependymoma. A follow-up study of 101 cases. *Cancer* 1977;40:907–15.

Palma L, Guidetti B. Cystic pilocytic astrocytomas of the cerebral hemispheres: surgical experience with 51 cases and long-term result. *J Neurosurg* 1985;62;811–15.

Yung WKA, Albright RE, J Olson et al. A phase II study of temozolomide versus procarbazine in patients with glioblastoma multiforme at first relapse. *Br J Cancer* 2000;85:588–93.

Yung WKA, Prados MD, Yaya-Tur P et al. Multicenter phase II trial of temozolomide in patients with anaplastic astrocytoma or anaplastic oligoastrocytomas at first relapse. *J Clin Oncol* 1999;17:2762–71.

Meningiomas are neoplasms that arise from the coverings of the brain and spinal cord, the meninges. The annual incidence of meningiomas is at least 2 per 100 000. They are the most common meningeal tumor and the most frequently encountered intracranial neoplasm. Meningiomas comprise approximately 20% of all brain tumors, and at least 90% are histologically benign or typical. However, a few are histologically atypical and aggressive, or frankly malignant.

The WHO classification of meningiomas is presented in Table 6.1. There are many histological subtypes of benign meningiomas. With the exception of the papillary meningioma, which tends to be particularly

TABLE 6.1

Modified World Health Organization classification of meningiomas

- Meningioma
  - Meningothelial
  - Fibrous (fibroblastic)
  - Transitional (mixed)
  - Psammomatous
  - Angiomatous
  - Microcystic
  - Secretory
  - Clear cell
  - Chordoid
  - Lymphoplasmacyte-rich
  - Metaplastic
- Atypical meningioma
- Papillary meningioma
- Anaplastic (malignant) meningioma

aggressive, these subtypes are descriptive and without prognostic significance.

Atypical meningiomas have frequent mitoses, large nuclei with prominent nucleoli, increased cellularity and necrosis. Malignant meningiomas have frankly malignant histological features, and invade blood vessels and brain.

Meningiomas are most frequently diagnosed in patients aged 50–80 years, and affect women 2–3 times as often as men (Table 6.2). Most patients present with seizures as their only symptom, and 10% have no symptoms at diagnosis.

The diagnosis of meningioma is suggested by the unique radiographic features (Figure 6.1). Meningiomas are isodense on unenhanced CT scans and isointense on unenhanced MRI scans; they enhance homogeneously when contrast is administered. This suggests a disrupted blood–brain barrier and intense vascularity. It is not possible to distinguish benign meningiomas reliably from atypical and malignant meningiomas on the basis of CT or MRI features.

Although most meningiomas are histologically benign, they cause considerable morbidity because they are often not completely resectable, or are progressive or recurrent. Nevertheless, benign meningiomas are associated with a median survival in excess of 10 years with treatment.

Because meningiomas are frequently asymptomatic and tend to occur in elderly patients, the decision to treat is often a controversial one. When patients are diagnosed with an asymptomatic meningioma

TABLE 6.2

Risk factors for the development of meningiomas

- Female gender
- Advancing age
- Cranial irradiation
- Trauma
- Neurofibromatosis type 2

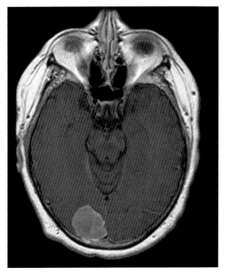

Figure 6.1 Contrast-enhanced axial MRI scan of a 55-year-old woman with a right occipital meningioma. The tumor abuts the sagittal sinus and probably arises from the falx. It is uniformly enhancing and, despite its size, produces no peritumoral edema.

by CT or MRI, a period of observation of up to 1 year is often suggested before a decision is taken to treat the tumor. The decision to delay treatment is based on the indolent and very long natural history of most meningiomas. For patients who have meningiomas that cause persistent neurological deficits, or for patients whose tumors have unusual radiographic features or are causing significant cerebral edema, an immediate intervention is often recommended.

Surgery

Surgery is the best treatment for meningiomas and the goal should be complete resection, whenever possible. Surgical complications include hemorrhage, new or worsened neurological deficits, and infections. However, complications are uncommon, even though many patients with meningiomas are elderly. Meningiomas that are completely resected are associated with recurrence rates of approximately 3% at 5 years and 20% at 20 years.

Meningiomas are highly vascular tumors, hence the blood supply must be coagulated before the tumor is removed by internal decompression. Usually, approximately 1 cm of dural attachment is removed with the tumor, as there is no distinct margin separating the meningioma from the dura. If CT or MRI demonstrates an enhancing dural tail, this should be removed with the tumor. A dural graft, usually pericranium, is used to repair the dural defect.

Meningiomas that involve the cerebral and cerebellar convexities can usually be completely removed. Those that arise from the falx usually produce leg weakness or seizures because they have a tendency to invade the superior sinus and are therefore difficult to manage surgically. It is best to remove as much tumor as possible without damaging the sinus. Observation and radiotherapy are the usual ways of dealing with residual tumor surrounding the sinus.

Unfortunately, many meningiomas, including those involving the skull base and cavernous sinus, are not completely resectable, even with the use of new surgical techniques such as subtemporal or transpetrosal approaches for tumors involving the anterior skull base or the petroclival region, respectively.

Skull base meningiomas are particularly difficult to manage because they usually invade dura and compress vital blood vessels and cranial nerves. In addition, they can become very large and extensive without causing substantial symptoms. Surgery is problematic because morbidity, usually in the form of new or worsened cranial nerve deficits, is in the range of 30–40% even in the best surgical hands. For such tumors located in inaccessible areas, aggressive surgical approaches that are likely to cause considerable and permanent morbidity are now often replaced by limited surgical resection combined with postoperative confocal radiotherapy. Similarly, optic nerve sheath meningiomas cannot be resected without sacrificing vision, and should therefore be treated with stereotactic radiotherapy if they are progressive.

Radiotherapy

Radiotherapy is becoming an increasingly important treatment option for meningiomas after initial subtotal resection or following recurrence. Radiotherapy appears to induce apoptosis in meningioma cells and consequently causes cessation of tumor growth, rather than tumor regression.

Improved technologies, such as conformal radiotherapy, stereotactic radiosurgery and stereotactic radiotherapy, limit the exposure of brain

Key points – meningiomas

- Meningiomas are the most common intracranial neoplasm. Most are low-grade and asymptomatic. Asymptomatic meningiomas may not require specific treatment, and can be observed by serial CT or MRI.
- Surgery is the principal therapeutic modality for symptomatic meningiomas, but many meningiomas cannot be completely resected because of their location in high-risk areas.
- Radiotherapy can achieve long-term growth stabilization of recurrent or enlarging meningiomas.

and tissues surrounding the meningioma to ionizing irradiation, thereby reducing the likelihood of radiation-induced injury. Nevertheless, single-dose radiosurgery is associated with significant complications, including cranial nerve injury and peritumoral edema. Conventional external beam radiotherapy also carries significant delayed toxicities, the most common of which is radiation-induced dementia. Despite these concerns, radiotherapy substantially delays time-to-recurrence for patients with meningiomas, with the most encouraging series reporting 10-year progression-free survival rates of 83% in patients who have undergone subtotal resection of benign meningiomas.

Medical therapy

There are limited therapeutic options for patients with meningiomas that are recurrent or progressive following maximal surgery and radiotherapy. Antiestrogenic and antiprogestational agents have been evaluated as potential treatments because meningiomas often express steroid receptors and the growth kinetics of some of these tumors are influenced by females sex hormones. However, these agents have no demonstrable efficacy.

Most trials have failed to show chemotherapeutic drugs to be effective for benign or malignant meningiomas. There has been recent interest in the use of hydroxyurea chemotherapy for benign meningiomas, with stabilization of enlarging benign meningiomas being observed in approximately 75% of patients treated for up to 2 years. Malignant meningiomas remain resistant to therapy, although a recent report has suggested a possible role for α-interferon in patients with such tumors.

Key references

Black PM. Meningiomas. *Neurosurgery* 1993;32:643–57.

Goldsmith BJ, Wara WM, Wilson CB, Larson DA. Postoperative irradiation for subtotally resected meningiomas. *J Neurosurg* 1994; 80:195–201.

Jaaskelainen J, Haltia M, Servo A. Atypical and anaplastic meningiomas: radiology, surgery, radiotherapy and outcome. *Surg Neurol* 1986;25:233–44.

Kondziolka D, Levy EI, Niranjan A et al. Long-term outcomes after meningioma radiosurgery: physician and patient outcomes. *J Neurosurg* 1999;91:44–50.

Mirimanoff RO, Dosoretz DE, Linggood RM et al. Meningioma: analysis of recurrence and progression following neurosurgical resection. *J Neurosurg* 1985;62: 18–24.

Petty AM, Kun LE, Meyer GA. Radiation therapy for incompletely resected meningiomas. *J Neurosurg* 1985;62:502–7.

Neuronal tumors are very uncommon brain neoplasms that preferentially affect children and young adults. There are often few signs and symptoms other than intractable epilepsy. The WHO classification of neuronal and mixed neuronal–glial tumors is shown in Table 7.1. The rarity of these neoplasms has been a source of considerable confusion and controversy, and it is only over the past two decades that many of these neoplasms have been recognized as distinct clinicopathological entities. General management guidelines are shown in Figure 7.1, and specific treatment issues are discussed below.

Gangliogliomas and gangliocytomas

Gangliogliomas consist of mature, well-differentiated but neoplastic ganglion cells within a normal neuropil. Gangliocytomas, in addition to having neoplastic ganglion cells, contain variable amounts of neoplastic glial cells, typically astrocytes. Despite these pathological differences, gangliogliomas and gangliocytomas have similar clinical and radiographic features. Although the vast majority of these tumors are

TABLE 7.1

World Health Organization classification of neuronal tumors

Tumor	Age at presentation (years)	Typical site
Ganglioglioma/gangliocytoma	< 30	Temporal lobe
Central neurocytoma	20–40	Intraventricular
Dysembryoplastic neuroepithelial tumor	< 30	Temporal lobe
Dysplastic gangliocytoma of the cerebellum	20–40	Cerebellum
Desmoplastic infantile ganglioglioma	< 2	Cerebral hemisphere

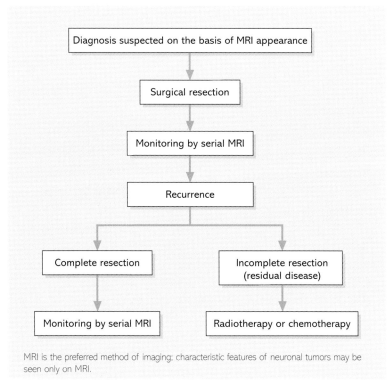

MRI is the preferred method of imaging; characteristic features of neuronal tumors may be seen only on MRI.

Figure 7.1 Management of neuronal tumors.

benign or low-grade, anaplastic variants and malignant degeneration of initially low-grade tumors have been described.

Gangliogliomas and gangliocytomas are uncommon, accounting for about 1.4% of all primary brain tumors, and typically present in patients under the age of 30 years. They have been reported at every site of the neuraxis, but most frequently in the temporal lobes. Epilepsy is the most common symptom because gangliogliomas and gangliocytomas both have a predilection for the cerebral hemispheres. All types of seizures may occur, including simple and complex partial seizures, and generalized seizures. When these tumors arise in other areas of the central nervous system they can produce a variety of symptoms, dependent on their location.

The CT and MRI features of gangliogliomas and gangliocytomas are striking. On CT scans, they appear as well-demarcated, cystic and partially calcified isodense masses that often enhance with contrast administration. MRI reveals a hypointense lesion with variable contrast enhancement on T1-weighted images, and a hyperintense lesion on T2-weighted images (Figure 7.2).

The initial management of gangliogliomas and gangliocytomas is surgery, with the goal of gross total resection of all accessible hemispheric tumors. If it is possible only to achieve incomplete resection, most authors recommend close observation with regular neuroimaging. Resection of these tumors can improve epilepsy, and approximately 68% of patients with epilepsy who undergo complete resection of their tumors become seizure-free.

The role of radiotherapy in managing these tumors is controversial. Some experts recommend radiotherapy for midline gangliogliomas and gangliocytomas and for tumors with an anaplastic glial element, based on retrospective data suggesting a worse outcome for these subsets of patients. Radiotherapy is also often administered at recurrence, but even in this situation, the initial approach is reoperation. There is no established role for chemotherapy, but agents used against gliomas are occasionally used to treat recurrent disease.

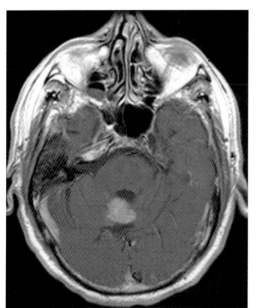

Figure 7.2 Contrast-enhanced axial magnetic resonance scan of a patient with a ganglioglioma involving the fourth ventricle. The lesion is uniformly enhancing, lacks calcifications and produces minimal peritumoral edema.

Central neurocytoma

Central neurocytoma was first described as a distinct entity in 1982. Previously, these tumors were classified as intraventricular oligodendrogliomas or intraventricular ependymomas. Histologically, central neurocytomas consist of uniform round cells that are positive for neuronal markers such as synaptophysin and neuron-specific enolase. In most cases, they are slow-growing neoplasms, but some tumors can be clinically aggressive.

Central neurocytomas constitute approximately 0.25% of all primary brain tumors. They are usually located between the hemispheres, attached either to the septum pellucidum or wall of the lateral ventricle. Rarely, they arise within the third ventricle or intraparenchymally. These tumors usually present in individuals aged 20–40 years. Symptoms are typically due to hydrocephalus, and include headaches, nausea and vomiting, and diplopia.

The radiographic appearance of central neurocytomas is characteristic (Figure 7.3). They are typically calcified, partially cystic isointense or hyperintense masses located in the anterior compartment of the ventricles, with variable contrast enhancement on T1- and T2-weighted MRI scans. Characteristically, the enhancing border of the tumor is sharply demarcated from the surrounding ventricles.

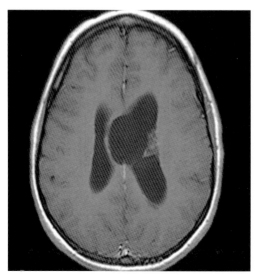

Figure 7.3 Contrast-enhanced T1-weighted MRI scan of a 26-year-old patient with a central neurocytoma. The lesion arises from the wall of the lateral ventricle, is multicystic and demonstrates moderate enhancement.

Complete surgical resection is required for central neurocytomas. No subsequent treatment is indicated immediately, but close clinical and radiographic monitoring is mandatory. If there is recurrence, reoperation is indicated and radiotherapy should be considered, particularly if the recurrence was rapid.

Dysplastic gangliocytoma of the cerebellum

Dysplastic gangliocytoma is a rare disorder combining neoplastic and malformative features. Macroscopically, megaloencephaly is a common finding, with the cerebellum demonstrating thickened folia. Microscopic examination of the cerebellum reveals disruption of cortical lamination by dysplastic neurons, and reduction or absence of white matter.

The disorder is usually diagnosed in individuals aged 10–40 years. The most common symptoms are those due to hydrocephalus and cerebellar dysfunction. Patients often have other malformations, including polydactyly and multiple hemangiomas. They may also suffer from seizures and mental retardation. An association with Cowden disease or multiple hamartoma syndrome has been reported, but the significance of this is uncertain.

MRI can reliably detect dysplastic gangliocytomas. T1- and T2-weighted images demonstrate a striated pattern of the cerebellar hemispheres corresponding to abnormally thickened cerebellar folia. Contrast enhancement is not a typical feature.

Radical resection of the mass lesion is the treatment of choice. In addition, ventriculoperitoneal shunting is often necessary for managing the symptoms of hydrocephalus. Although resection is often subtotal, persistence of a residual lesion may not adversely affect outcome. This lesion is very indolent, and there is no established role for radiotherapy or chemotherapy.

Dysembryoplastic neuroepithelial tumor

Dysembryoplastic neuroepithelial tumor is a rare and recently described entity that comprises a dysplastic mass of bundles of axons, surrounded by oligodendrocytes and neurons suspended in an interstitial fluid. There can be nodules of neoplastic oligodendrocytes and astrocytes, which can make pathological differentiation from gliomas difficult.

These lesions have combined hamartomatous and neoplastic characteristics, and are frequently located in temporal lobes. They have been identified in individuals of various ages, although most patients present in early childhood with epilepsy. There may be a slight male preponderance.

MRI reveals a cortically situated and well-demarcated lesion that is hypointense on T1-weighted images and hyperintense on T2-weighted images. Enhancement with contrast administration is uncommon; when present, it can be diffuse or patchy.

Surgical resection of the lesion is the only indicated treatment and, in the vast majority of patients, this cures the epileptic seizures. There is no role for radiotherapy or chemotherapy, as recurrence or malignant transformation has yet to be reported for this disorder.

Desmoplastic infantile ganglioglioma

Desmoplastic infantile gangliogliomas have solid and cystic components. Microscopically, they can be seen to consist of neoplastic neurons and astrocytes surrounded by a dense desmoplastic reaction. This type of tumor is very rare, with only a few dozen cases having been reported to date, all in infants and young children. There appears to be a male predominance.

Patients typically present with an enlarged head and other features of hydrocephalus, and also seizures. These tumors are confined to the cerebral hemispheres, and MRI usually reveals a massive multicystic

---

Key points – neuronal tumors

- Neuronal tumors are uncommon brain neoplasms typically diagnosed in children and young adults.
- The principal management of neuronal tumors is surgical; total or subtotal resection can be associated with long-term tumor control.
- The behavior of these tumors can be unpredictable and remains poorly understood because of their rarity.

multilobulated mass with a solid component extending to the cortical surface. Enhancement with contrast is often seen within the solid elements and, rarely, in the walls of the cystic components.

As with all glial–neuronal tumors, initial management comprises maximal surgical resection of the tumor. Subsequent management is not clear. Postoperative chemotherapy or radiotherapy has often been administered following subtotal resection, because the tumor has the potential for aggressive biological behavior. For patients undergoing macroscopically radical resections, further immediate therapy can be withheld because the prognosis associated with this tumor is usually good.

Key references

Dumas-Duport C, Scheithauer JP, Chodkiewicz ER et al. Dysembryoplastic neuroepithelial tumor: a surgically curable tumor of young patients with intractable partial seizures. Report of thirty-nine cases. *Neurosurgery* 1988;23: 545–56.

Krouwer HG, Davis RL, McDermott MW et al. Ganglioglioma: a clinicopathological study of 25 cases and review of the literature. *J Neurooncol* 1993;17:139–54.

Lang FF, Epstein FJ, Ransohoff J. Central nervous system ganglioglioma. 2: Clinical outcome. *J Neurosurg* 1993;79:867–73.

Padberg GW, Schot JDL, Vielvoye GJ et al. Lhermitte–Duclos disease and Cowden disease: a single phakomatosis. *Ann Neurol* 1991;29: 517–23.

Schild SE, Scheithauer BW, Haddock MG et al. Central neurocytomas. *Cancer* 1997;79:790–5.

Vandenberg SR, May EE, Rubinstein LJ et al. Desmoplastic supratentorial neuroepithelial tumors of infancy with divergent differentiation potential ('desmoplastic infantile gangliogliomas'). *J Neurosurg* 1987;66:58–71.

Vinchon M, Blond S, Lejeune JP et al. Association of Lhermitte–Duclos and Cowden disease: report of a new case and a review of the literature. *J Neurol Neurosurg Psychiatry* 1994;57:699–704.

Yasargil MG, von Ammon K, Von Deimling A et al. Central neurocytoma: histopathological variants and therapeutic approaches. *J Neurosurg* 1992;76:32–7.

Pineal region tumors present with characteristic symptoms and signs, which depend on tumor location. The most common presenting sign is obstructive hydrocephalus, due to occlusion of the aqueduct of Sylvius. Compression of the superior colliculus causes Parinaud syndrome, with limited upgaze, light-near dissociation of pupillary response and convergence–retraction nystagmus. Compression of the superior cerebellar peduncles may result in dysmetria or ataxia. Pineal apoplexy (i.e. sudden hemorrhage at the tumor site) may cause acute visual loss, diplopia or loss of consciousness.

It is useful to consider pineal region tumors as a group for the purposes of differential diagnosis. The tumors in this region include germ cell tumors, pineal parenchymal tumors, pineal region cysts, gliomas, meningiomas and Vein of Galen aneurysms (Table 8.1). The wide range of tumor types that can arise in the pineal region make histological diagnosis mandatory. The only exception is a patient with elevated CSF markers that indicate the presence of a malignant germ cell tumor.

Germ cell tumors

Germ cell tumors, the most common type of tumor in the pineal region, comprise a heterogeneous group of primary brain tumors arising from pluripotential germinal cells. The most common is the germinoma, accounting for 40–60% of all germ cell tumors. Other germ cell tumors include teratomas, and non-germinomatous germ cell tumors such as choriocarcinoma, endodermal sinus tumor and embryonal carcinoma. The different germ cell tumor markers are shown in Table 8.2.

In the Western hemisphere, these tumors account for 0.4–3.4% of intracranial neoplasms. For unknown reasons, the incidence in Japan is significantly higher at 2.1–9.4%, and non-germinomatous germ cell tumors constitute an increased proportion of all germ cell tumors.

More than 70% of germ cell tumors present before the patient reaches the age of 21 years, typically in those aged 10–13 years. Most

TABLE 8.1

Differential diagnosis of a pineal region mass

- Pineal parenchymal tumor
- Germ cell tumor
- Meningioma
- Tectal astrocytoma
- Vein of Galen aneurysm
- Dermoid/epidermoid cyst
- Pineal cyst

TABLE 8.2

Germ cell tumor markers

	AFP	β-HCG	PAP
Germinomas	–	±	+
Non-germinomatous germ cell tumor			
Choriocarcinoma	–	+	±
Embryonal carcinoma	–	–	+
Endodermal sinus (yolk sac) tumor	+	–	±
Teratoma			
Mature	–		–
Immature	±	–	+

AFP, α–fetoprotein; β-HCG, human chorionic gonadotropin; PAP, placental alkaline phosphatase

arise in the pineal region, but one-third occur in the suprasellar region. Males are 2–4 times more likely than females to develop a germ cell tumor, but there is a predilection for suprasellar tumors to occur in females. An increased incidence of germ cell tumors has been reported in both Klinefelter and Down syndrome.

Pathology. Germinomas are composed of large round cells with vesicular nuclei and granular eosinophilic cytoplasm. These cells stain for placental alkaline phosphatase, which may also be detected in the serum and cerebrospinal fluid (CSF). A small number of germinomas harbor syncytiotrophoblastic giant cells.

Non-germinomatous germ cell tumors are highly malignant and commonly exhibit mixed histological features. Embryonal carcinomas arise from pluripotent embryonic epithelial cells and rarely occur in pure form. Endodermal sinus or yolk sac tumors arise from the extraembryonic yolk sac endoderm; cytoplasmic and extracellular droplets immunoreactive for α-fetoprotein are diagnostic. Choriocarcinomas are composed of bilaminar trophoblastic cells with high levels of β-human chorionic gonadotrophin (β-HCG) and are prone to spontaneous hemorrhage.

Teratomas are most common in infants and very young children and are divided into mature and immature types. Mature teratomas are made up of fully differentiated tissues and are benign. Immature teratomas are much more common than mature teratomas, and may have elements of carcinoma, sarcoma or other non-germinomatous germ cell tumors.

Clinical features. Patients with pineal region tumors present with features of obstructive hydrocephalus, resulting from occlusion of the aqueduct of Sylvius. Compression of the superior colliculus causes Parinaud syndrome with limited upgaze, light-near dissociation of pupillary response and convergence–retraction nystagmus. Dysmetria or ataxia may result from compression of the superior cerebellar peduncles.

In addition to tumors in the pineal region, a subset of germ cell tumors arise in a suprasellar location. Suprasellar tumors have visual and endocrine manifestations, including diabetes insipidus, growth failure and precocious puberty. Ninety percent of postpubertal girls with these tumors develop secondary amenorrhea, and 33% of prepubertal girls have growth arrest. Males with choriocarcinoma have a 50% incidence of precocious puberty. Decreased visual acuity occurs in up to 84% of patients. Local invasion of the thalamus may result in hemiparesis.

Diagnostic criteria. The are various means of evaluating a suspected germ cell tumor, as shown in Table 8.3. The gold standard for diagnosis is histopathology. This mandates a surgical biopsy, preferably open as opposed to stereotactic biopsy to ensure adequate sampling. This is particularly important when a non-germinomatous germ cell tumor is suspected, as these tumors often have mixed histology. Prognosis and treatment are determined by the most malignant histology within a tumor.

The only circumstance in which histopathology is not mandatory for diagnosis is when a patient has elevated CSF markers that indicate the presence of a malignant germ cell tumor.

Although serum and CSF markers can be helpful when positive, negative markers do not exclude an aggressive histology, as non-germinomatous germ cell tumors can be marker-negative. CSF α-fetoprotein signals the presence of primitive yolk sac elements, indicative of endodermal sinus tumor. β-HCG points to the presence of primitive placental cells and is markedly elevated in choriocarcinoma; it may be slightly elevated (< 50 mIU/mL) in pure germinomas with a syncytiotrophoblastic element. Other markers have been reported but are less specific and therefore less helpful. The CSF should be sampled for cytology and markers at the time of ventriculoperitoneal shunt placement or at least 2 weeks after debulking surgery.

TABLE 8.3

Evaluation of a newly diagnosed or suspected germ cell tumor

- MRI brain scanning with gadolinium
- MRI total spine scanning with gadolinium (except mature teratoma)
- Serum and CSF levels of AFP and β-HCG*
- CSF cytology*
- Endocrine evaluation
- Formal visual field testing (sellar or suprasellar tumors)

*If hydrocephalus is present, CSF should be obtained at time of shunt or third ventriculostomy
CSF, cerebrospinal fluid; AFP, α-fetoprotein; β-HCG, β-human chorionic gonadotropin

Neuroimaging characteristics may suggest the diagnosis. Germinomas tend to be homogeneous and isointense to white matter on T1-weighted MRI and slightly hyperintense on T2-weighted images. Gadolinium enhancement is intense and uniform (Figure 8.1). Teratomas and non-germinomatous germ cell tumors are notably

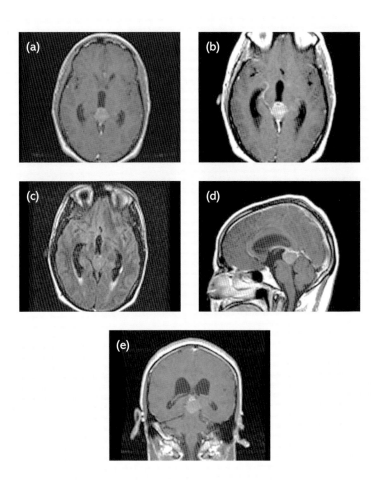

Figure 8.1 Multiple MRI sequences of a pineal region germinoma in a 29-year-old man. (a) Precontrast hyperintensity of this cellular tumor; (b) dense contrast enhancement and (c) isointensity of this lesion on fluid-attenuated inversion-recovery (FLAIR) scans. (d) Sagittal and (e) coronal images illustrate the boundaries of the pineal region.

heterogeneous on MRI, both pre- and post-contrast, and are more likely than pure germinomas to show evidence of infiltration into surrounding normal brain. Areas of previous hemorrhage are typical of choriocarcinoma (Figure 8.2).

Although characteristic neuroimaging findings may suggest a particular diagnosis, definitive pathology should always be obtained. CSF studies and spinal MRI should also be obtained in all patients with a germ cell tumor.

Treatment differs for pure germinomas, teratomas and non-germinomatous germ cell tumors, as described below.

Surgical resection is not indicated for pure germinomas. However, other germ cell tumors benefit from radical resection and mature teratomas can be cured with complete resection. Second-look surgery may be important in patients with apparent residual tumor following treatment, as this may represent an element of mature teratoma or necrosis that can be cured with resection.

Radiotherapy is the treatment of choice for patients with pure germinoma. The standard approach is to administer focal radiotherapy to the ventricular system at a dose of 40 Gy, followed by an additional 15 Gy to the tumor bed. Craniospinal radiation is mandated if there is evidence of leptomeningeal dissemination on CSF cytology or contrast-enhanced spinal MRI. The use of craniospinal radiotherapy has been recommended for all patients by some experts, to decrease

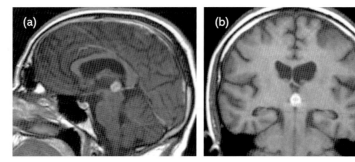

Figure 8.2 Gadolinium-enhanced T1-weighted (a) sagittal and (b) coronal images of a non-germinomatous germ cell tumor, predominantly choriocarcinoma, in a 24-year-old man.

the risk of leptomeningeal relapse. Other experts recommend using lower or more focused doses of radiotherapy to avoid delayed radiation toxicity.

Chemotherapy. All germ cell tumors are chemosensitive and successful regimens, usually platinum-based, have been reported for relapse, adjuvant and neoadjuvant treatment. As patients with pure germinoma can anticipate an excellent outcome with radiotherapy alone (5-year survival up to 95%), the use of chemotherapy alone should be confined to carefully selected patients in clinical trials (e.g. it might be trialed in young patients to minimize potential cognitive toxicity by avoiding radiotherapy). Ideally, patients with non-germinomatous germ cell tumors should be treated within a clinical trial; otherwise, they should receive 2–6 cycles of platinum-based chemotherapy prior to radiotherapy.

Symptomatic therapy. Patients presenting with hydrocephalus require ventricular decompression. This can be accomplished by ventriculoperitoneal shunt placement, third ventriculostomy or tumor debulking. Ventriculoperitoneal shunt placement is the most frequently used method, but there are reports of secondary intraperitoneal metastases. Therefore, endoscopic third ventriculostomy may be preferable.

Suprasellar tumors may present with a variety of endocrinological syndromes. Endocrine dysfunction, including hypopituitarism and diabetes insipidus, may also develop after radiotherapy. Therefore, it is recommended that all patients with suprasellar germ cell tumors be evaluated and followed by an endocrinologist.

Long-term outcome. Germ cell tumors tend to recur locally. Leptomeningeal recurrence is usually accompanied by recurrence at the primary tumor site. Distant metastases to bone and lung have been reported, but are uncommon. At recurrence, treatment is often limited by the choice of prior therapy, but potential options include reoperation, radiosurgery and salvage chemotherapy.

Delayed complications of radiotherapy are a significant concern. Long-term survivors are at risk of cognitive deficits, hypothalamic and endocrine dysfunction, and radiation-induced neoplasms. Careful attention should be paid to school performance to identify and treat learning disabilities. Vigilant monitoring of endocrine function may minimize disability. Treatment-induced brain malignancy should be considered in all patients with an apparent late radiographic recurrence.

Pineal parenchymal tumors

Pineal parenchymal tumors can be divided into low (pineocytoma), intermediate (pineal parenchymal) and high (pineoblastoma) grade. Pineocytomas typically occur in adults and can be cured with surgical resection; radiotherapy or stereotactic radiosurgery should be used in patients with an incomplete resection. Pineoblastomas typically occur in children and young adults; when seen in conjunction with familial retinoblastoma, these are called trilateral retinoblastoma.

Pineoblastomas are highly malignant tumors with a predilection to leptomeningeal dissemination (Figure 8.3). CSF studies and spinal MRI should be carried out in all patients with pineoblastoma. Patients should be treated with chemotherapy and craniospinal radiotherapy, with a focal boost to the tumor site.

Intermediate-grade tumors, sometimes referred to as mixed pineocytoma–pineoblastoma, have an unpredictable growth rate and clinical behavior.

Treatment of pineal region tumors is summarized in Table 8.4.

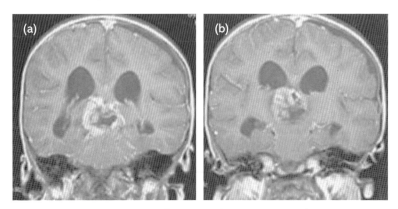

Figure 8.3 Gadolinium-enhanced T1-weighted coronal images of a large irregularly enhancing pineoblastoma in a 3-year-old child. The tumor has caused secondary obstructive hydrocephalus with enlargement of the lateral ventricles and prominent temporal horns. Image (a) is slightly anterior to image (b).

TABLE 8.4

Treatment of pineal region tumors

Surgery
- Meningioma
- Mature teratoma
- Pineal parenchymal tumors
- Consider second-look surgery in non-germinomatous germ cell tumor

Radiotherapy
- Germinoma
- Incompletely resected pineocytoma

Chemotherapy + radiotherapy
- Non-germinomatous germ cell tumor
- Pineoblastoma

Pineal region cysts

Pineal parenchymal cysts are asymptomatic incidental lesions found on MRI scanning. Occasional cysts larger than 15 mm will cause symptomatic hydrocephalus or other neurological findings. Epidermoid and dermoid cysts may also occur in the pineal region.

Key points – pineal region tumors

- Tumors of the pineal region often present with obstructive hydrocephalus.
- The wide range of tumor types that can arise in the pineal region make histological diagnosis mandatory. The only exception is a patient with elevated CSF markers that indicate the presence of a malignant germ cell tumor.
- CSF studies and spinal MRI should be obtained in all patients with a germ cell tumor or pineoblastoma.

Key references

Balmaceda C, Heller G, Rosenblum M et al. Chemotherapy without irradiation – a novel approach for newly diagnosed CNS germ cell tumors: results of an international cooperative trial. The First International Central Nervous System Germ Cell Tumor Study. *J Clin Oncol* 1996;14:2908–15.

Kondziolka D, Hadjipanayis CG, Flickinger JC, Lunsford LD. The role of radiosurgery for the treatment of pineal parenchymal tumors. *Neurosurgery* 2002;51:880–9.

Lutterbach J, Fauchon F, Schild SE et al. Malignant pineal parenchymal tumors in adult patients: patterns of care and prognostic factors. *Neurosurgery* 2002;51:44–55, discussion 55–6.

Nakamura M, Saeki N, Iwadate Y et al. Neuroradiological characteristics of pineocytoma and pineoblastoma. *Neuroradiology* 2000;42:509–14.

Tamaki N, Yin D. Therapeutic strategies and surgical results for pineal region tumors. *J Clin Neurosci* 2000;7:125–8.

Wolden SL, Wara WM, Larson DA et al. Radiation therapy for primary intracranial germ-cell tumors. *Int J Radiat Oncol Biol Phys* 1995;32:943–9.

Skull base tumors are neoplasms that arise from or involve the skull base. These tumors pose a surgical challenge because of their deep location within the cranium and close proximity to critical neurovascular structures. Recently, advances in neuroimaging, improved surgical tools and techniques, and new methods of stereotactically focusing radiotherapy have improved the prognosis in patients with cranial base tumors.

Symptoms of skull base tumors arise from involvement of cranial nerves, compression of brainstem or basal cerebral structures, and obstruction of the pharynx, middle ear or nasal cavity.

This chapter reviews the most common primary skull base tumors and discusses general principles of management. Meningiomas and pituitary adenomas are addressed in Chapters 6 and 10.

Classification

Skull base tumors can be classified according to their location or biological behavior. The location of a skull base tumor strongly influences clinical presentation, differential diagnosis and management. Table 9.1 lists the important tumors arising from specific regions of the skull base. Pathologically, skull base tumors can be classified as benign, of intermediate malignancy or highly malignant. A classification of skull base tumors by biological behavior is presented in Table 9.2.

Diagnostic tests

MRI is the imaging modality of choice for all skull base neoplasms because it is accurate in providing tumor dimensions and location, as well as in depicting critical vascular structures such as the carotid and vertebrobasilar arteries and branches. Magnetic resonance angiography has largely replaced intra-arterial angiography as a means of obtaining detailed information about the vascular architecture around the tumor. Nevertheless, conventional angiography still provides useful and precise information about tumor vasculature, and offers an opportunity for

TABLE 9.1

Tumors arising from specific regions of the skull base

Anterior cranial base

- Meningioma
- Esthesioneuroblastoma
- Nasopharyngeal carcinoma

Middle cranial base

- Meningioma
- Pituitary adenoma
- Craniopharyngioma
- Schwannoma
- Adenoid cystic carcinoma
- Chordoma

Posterior cranial base

- Meningioma
- Schwannoma
- Chordoma
- Chondrosarcoma
- Dermoid cyst
- Epidermoid cyst
- Paraganglioma

TABLE 9.2

Skull base tumors classified by biological behavior

Benign

- Meningioma
- Schwannoma
- Pituitary adenoma
- Paraganglioma
- Epidermoid cyst
- Dermoid cyst

Intermediate malignancy

- Adenoid cystic carcinoma
- Chordoma
- Chondrosarcoma
- Low-grade esthesioneuroblastoma

High malignancy

- Primary sarcoma
- Skull base carcinoma
- Skull base lymphoma
- High-grade esthesioneuroblastoma

preoperative embolization of the vascular supply of highly vascular tumors, which can reduce intraoperative blood loss and time. CT scans are especially useful for delineating bony structures and destruction, and intratumoral calcifications. Using these imaging techniques, it is often possible to diagnose skull base tumors preoperatively with considerable certainty.

Management

The management options for skull base tumors are surgery, radiotherapy or chemotherapy, or combinations thereof, or careful observation with close follow-up. For skull base tumors that are benign, and causing minimal symptoms and signs, observation is often recommended because surgical intervention may cause considerable morbidity. Histological confirmation of a diagnosis can be deferred if imaging studies are characteristic of a benign neoplasm with a favorable natural history, such as a meningioma. However, regular follow-up with imaging is then necessary to monitor tumor progression.

The decision to operate must be made on an individual basis, depending on the likelihood of benefit from tumor resection. Hence, surgery is most often offered to patients with progressive symptoms. It can be curative if benign skull base tumors are resected completely. Modern skull base surgery incorporates removal of non-critical skull base bone and has provided excellent access to deep-seated tumors, with reduced cerebral retraction. Consequently, it is now possible to carry out more radical surgery, with reduced morbidity. However, there are still risks associated with surgery, including cranial neuropathies, infections and CSF leak.

A number of radiotherapeutic modalities have been used to control tumor growth of skull base neoplasms with reasonable success and minimal complications. Conventional fractionated radiotherapy has been used to control benign tumors such as meningiomas and paraganglogliomas, as well as to provide palliative treatment for malignant tumors. Promising results have been obtained for relatively radioresistant tumors such as chordomas and chondrosarcomas with particle-beam therapy. Stereotactic radiosurgery is being used increasingly for small tumors, such as schwannomas or small meningiomas, in surgically high-risk areas, with promising results (Figure 9.1).

Chemotherapy has a very limited role in the management of most skull base tumors, but is incorporated in the treatment of chemosensitive neoplasms such as esthesioneuroblastoma, skull base lymphoma and nasopharyngeal carcinoma.

Specific tumors

Schwannomas account for 6–8% of all intracranial tumors. The natural history of these tumors is favorable, and small asymptomatic schwannomas are usually managed with close observation. Vestibular schwannomas (acoustic neuromas) are the most common type, but schwannomas can develop from other cranial nerves such as the trigeminal or facial nerve. Symptoms relate to dysfunction of the involved cranial nerve. Typical symptoms in patients with vestibular schwannomas are tinnitus and impaired hearing.

In most cases, schwannomas are managed surgically. The goal is to achieve total resection of tumor with preservation of cranial nerve

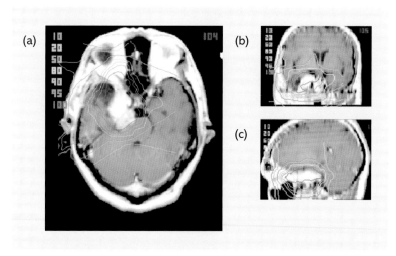

Figure 9.1 Stereotactic radiotherapy plan for a patient with a cavernous sinus meningioma. Dose distributions in (a) axial, (b) coronal and (c) sagittal planes demonstrate how this technique delivers therapeutic doses of radiotherapy to an irregular tumor while largely sparing normal surrounding structures.

function. In the case of vestibular schwannomas, the facial nerve remains at risk, but modern surgical techniques can preserve nerve function in the vast majority of cases. Stereotactic radiosurgery is an increasingly attractive alternative for patients with schwannomas, and has been shown to control tumor growth in as many as 97% of cases, although follow-up has been short. Larger tumor size is associated with increased surgical morbidity, and increased risk of radiotherapeutic failure.

A minority of schwannomas, including bilateral vestibular schwannomas, is associated with neurofibromatosis type II. Schwannomas that are associated with this disorder are reported to be more aggressive and invasive than sporadic tumors.

Paragangliomas arise from paraganglion tissue in the head and neck. Paragangliomas of the brain arise from the glomus tympanicum in the middle ear, and the glomus jugulare at the jugular base. Presenting symptoms are most commonly tinnitus or hearing loss, or vocal cord dysfunction. These tumors develop more commonly in women, and can arise at any age. Multiple tumors or a familial occurrence is noted in 10% of cases.

Surgery and radiotherapy are the principal approaches to management. Complete resection is curative, and can be achieved in almost all glomus tympanicum tumors and in as many as 80% of glomus jugulare tumors. Radiotherapy can control most tumors when there is recurrence or tumor progression following surgery.

Esthesioneuroblastomas are rare tumors arising from the basal cells of the olfactory epithelium (Figure 9.2). Presenting symptoms include epistaxis and nasal congestion. A minority of patients have CNS symptoms. Esthesioneuroblastomas can be slow-growing tumors, but their behavior is unpredictable.

Surgery with or without postoperative radiotherapy appears to confer the best outcome. Multiple-agent chemotherapy may improve the outcome in some patients, such as those with postoperative residual disease or with tumors of high pathological grade.

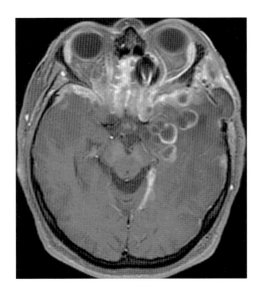

Figure 9.2 Contrast-enhanced T1-weighted axial image demonstrating extensive esthesioneuroblastoma involving sinuses, skull base and leptomeninges, with invasion into adjacent temporal lobes.

Esthesioneuroblastomas may recur after long disease-free intervals, necessitating prolonged follow-up. Recurrences are usually local, but regional lymph node and distant metastases are not uncommon.

Chordomas and chondrosarcomas are uncommon tumors arising from bone. Preoperative differentiation between these tumors on the basis of imaging features is difficult, although chordomas are often situated centrally and chondrosarcomas laterally at the skull base. Chordomas may show areas of high signal, representing gelatinous areas, on T1-weighted images.

Intracranial chordomas arise from the clivus and account for fewer than 1% of all intracranial tumors. Typical presenting symptoms are diplopia and headache. These tumors are managed with surgery and radiotherapy. Maximal surgical resection and younger age are associated with longer disease-free survival.

Chondrosarcomas can be subgrouped into myxochondrosarcomas and mesenchymal or embryonal chondrosarcomas. They typically arise in the middle of the cranial fossa, with extension to the posterior cranial fossa. Chondrosarcomas are more surgically accessible than chordomas and also arise in younger patients. These factors may contribute to the better overall prognosis for patients with chondrosarcoma. Five-year recurrence-free survival rates have been reported as 90% for patients with chondrosarcomas, and 65% for those with chordomas.

Key points – skull base tumors

- Symptoms of tumors of the skull base arise from involvement of cranial nerves, compression of brainstem or basal cerebral structures, and obstruction of the pharynx, middle ear or nasal cavity.
- Surgery can be curative if benign skull base tumors are resected completely. However, there is a relatively high risk of operative morbidity.
- Radiosurgery is an increasingly accepted alternative to surgery for small tumors in surgically high-risk areas.
- Particle-beam radiation can achieve long-term control of growth for radioresistant skull base tumors such as chordomas and chondrosarcomas.

Key references

Cusimano MD, Sekhar LN, Sen CN et al. The results of surgery for benign tumors of the cavernous sinus. *Neurosurgery* 1995;37:1–9.

Ebersold MJ, Morita A, Olsen KD et al. Glomus jugulare tumors. In : Kaye AH, Laws ER, eds. *Brain Tumors*. Edinburgh: Churchill Livingstone, 1995:795–807.

Eden BV, Debo RF, Larner JM et al. Esthesioneuroblastoma: long-term outcome and patterns of failure – the University of Virginia experience. *Cancer* 1994;73:2556–62.

Forsyth PA, Cascino TL, Shaw EG et al. Intracranial chordomas: a clinicopathological and prognostic study of 51 cases. *J Neurosurg* 1993;78:741–7.

Matthies C. Management of 1000 vestibular schwannomas (acoustic neuromas): clinical presentation. *Neurosurgery* 1997;40:1–10.

Sammi M, Migliori MM, Tatagliba M et al. Surgical treatment of trigeminal schwannomas. *J Neurosurg* 1995;82:711–18.

Sammi M. Management of 1000 vestibular schwannomas (acoustic neuromas): surgical management and results with an emphasis on complications and how to avoid them. *Neurosurgery* 1997;40:11–23.

Sekkhar LN, Moller AR. Operative management of tumors involving the cavernous sinus. *J Neurosurg* 1986; 64:879–89.

Pituitary adenomas are the third most common type of primary intracranial tumors (after gliomas and meningiomas), accounting for 10–15% of all such tumors. Improvements in neuroimaging increasingly reveal incidental, usually asymptomatic, pituitary adenomas. These occult microadenomas have been reported on as many as 10–15% of routine MRIs.

Multiple endocrine neoplasia type 1 (MEN-1) is an autosomal dominant disorder associated with tumors of the parathyroid, pancreatic islet cells and pituitary. Patients with MEN-1 have about a 25% risk of developing a pituitary adenoma, usually a macroadenoma that secretes growth hormone or prolactin.

Pituitary adenomas may present clinically with endocrinological or neurological dysfunction, or both. Most patients are diagnosed between the ages of 20 and 60 years; younger patients are more likely to have a tumor that actively secretes a hormone. Approximately 70% of pituitary adenomas secrete a hormone, and thus present with an endocrine abnormality. In addition, macroadenomas (tumors larger than 1 cm in diameter) may present with signs and symptoms of pituitary insufficiency secondary to compression of the pituitary stalk or gland.

Headache is the most common neurological symptom. Patients are also at risk of visual loss secondary to compression of the optic chiasm; this classically presents with a bitemporal hemianopia, but the presentation is often asymmetrical or atypical.

Pituitary apoplexy is a rare neurological presentation of a pituitary tumor, in which there is acute development of headache, visual loss, ophthalmoplegia, altered level of consciousness, and cardiovascular collapse secondary to adrenal failure. This syndrome occurs as a result of intratumoral hemorrhage or acute necrosis with edema and compression. This presentation constitutes a medical emergency; patients require stress doses of glucocorticoids and urgent surgical decompression.

Endocrinological consultation can be invaluable in the precise delineation and care of patients with pituitary adenoma. Baseline evaluation should include: prolactin, growth hormone, adrenocorticotropic hormone (ACTH), luteinizing hormone (LH), follicle-stimulating hormone (FSH), thyroid-stimulating hormone (TSH), thyroxine, cortisol, insulin-like growth factor 1 (IGF-1), testosterone and estradiol. Additional tests or specific attempts at hormone stimulation may be important in defining specific syndromes.

MRI is the procedure of choice for imaging the pituitary region (Figure 10.1). Microadenomas are defined as tumors up to 1 cm in diameter and macroadenomas are those greater than 1 cm. CT may be useful to evaluate hemorrhage in the setting of pituitary apoplexy. It may also help to identify the extent of bony destruction associated with a macroadenoma, or to identify hyperostosis that may be seen with a pituitary meningioma.

Pathologically, pituitary adenomas are classified using immunohistochemistry to define the hormone secreted. Earlier systems of classification based on cytoplasmic staining (i.e. acidophilic, basophilic, chromophobic) are no longer used. Most adenomas appear histologically benign, and atypical or aggressive features (e.g. necrosis, increased cellularity) do not have clear clinical implications.

Disorders to be considered in the differential diagnosis of a sellar mass are listed in Table 10.1. The goals of therapy are to reverse

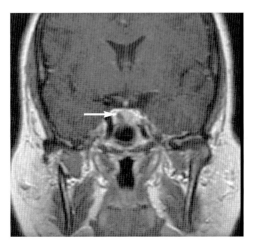

Figure 10.1 Gadolinium-enhanced T1-weighted MRI of the sella, demonstrating a non-secreting pituitary adenoma (arrow) in a 54-year-old woman.

TABLE 10.1

Differential diagnosis of a sellar mass

- Pituitary adenoma
- Pituitary metastases/lymphoma
- Germ cell tumor
- Craniopharyngioma
- Optic nerve/chiasm glioma
- Rathke cleft cyst
- Meningioma
- Carotid aneurysm
- Langerhans cell histiocytosis
- Lymphocytic hypophysitis
- Granuloma
- Sarcoidosis
- Abscess

endocrinopathy, to eliminate mass effects with preservation or restoration of neurological function (particularly vision), and to prevent recurrence. Specific tumor types are discussed below, and Table 10.2 summarizes treatment for pituitary adenomas.

Prolactinomas

Prolactinomas are the most common subtype of pituitary adenomas, accounting for 30% of these tumors (Figure 10.2). In addition to the classic syndrome of amenorrhea/galactorrhea, patients often experience decreased libido, dyspareunia and headache. There is a significant risk of osteoporosis as a result of hypogonadism.

Prolactin levels seen in association with a secreting adenoma are usually in excess of 200 ng/mL; levels in excess of 1000 ng/mL are indicative of invasive tumor. Moderate elevations of prolactin (20–150 ng/mL) may be seen with other pituitary adenomas as a result of pituitary stalk compression. Other medical conditions may also cause moderate prolactinemia (Table 10.3).

Medical management with a dopamine agonist (bromocriptine or cabergoline) is successful in normalizing prolactin levels, preserving fertility and decreasing tumor size in 50–100% of patients. Patients with microadenomas are particularly likely to respond well to medical treatment. However, lifelong therapy is required because most patients will have recurrent symptoms and tumor growth if the dopamine

TABLE 10.2

Treatment of pituitary adenomas

Surgery – 96% transphenoidal

- Treatment of choice for pituitary adenomas other than prolactinomas
- Control of progressive mass effect/neurological symptoms
- Failed medical therapy (usually patients with prolactinoma)
- Diagnosis (if tissue diagnosis is mandatory), enabling treatment to be planned
- Pituitary apoplexy (constitutes a neurosurgical emergency; operation proceeds as soon as patient is medically stable)

Medical management

- Dopamine agonists (bromocriptine, cabergoline)
  - Prolactinomas
  - Other pituitary adenomas with moderate prolactinemia
  - GH secretors
- Somatostatin analogs (octreotide, lanreotide)
  - Growth hormone secreters, up to 60% response reported
  - Refractory TSH-secreting pituitary adenomas
- Mitotane, ketoconazole, metyrapone and DVT prophylaxis may each be given alone or in combination
  - Cushing disease

Radiotherapy

- Recurrent or refractory tumors
- Large invasive tumors
  - Inoperable
  - Incomplete resection with persistent symptoms

agonist is discontinued. Surgery is appropriate for patients with resistant tumors and for those unable to tolerate medical therapy, or simply because of patient preference. Surgery is also undertaken to allow pregnancy without risk of tumor growth and to avoid the unknown risk to the fetus associated with the use of medication.

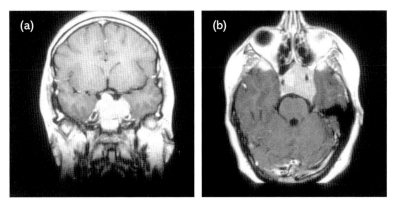

Figure 10.2 Gadolinium-enhanced T1-weighted images of a large prolactinoma in a 23-year-old woman. (a) Axial and (b) coronal images.

GH-secreting pituitary adenomas

GH-secreting pituitary adenomas are insidious tumors that often present in slightly older patients and are more likely to be larger than 1 cm in diameter at the time of diagnosis. Signs and symptoms of acromegaly have often been present for nearly a decade prior to diagnosis. Growth hormone levels are above 5 ng/mL and most patients also have elevated IGF-1; in 40–50% of patients there is a modest elevation of prolactin.

Surgery is the initial treatment of choice. Medical management using somatostatin analogs such as octreotide are also effective. Radiotherapy may be necessary in patients with recurrent or refractory tumors.

TABLE 10.3

Causes of moderate prolactin elevation

- Stalk effect
- Drugs
  - Phenothiazines
  - Metoclopramide
  - Verapamil
  - Cimetidine
- Chronic renal failure
- Cirrhosis
- Hypothyroidism

ACTH-secreting pituitary adenomas

ACTH-secreting pituitary adenomas, accounting for 8–10% of all pituitary adenomas, represent the greatest endocrinological challenge. Definitive diagnosis depends on establishing a diagnosis of Cushing disease on the basis of hormone parameters (Table 10.4) and excluding ectopic sources of ACTH secretion (Table 10.5). Women are affected 3–10 times more often than men, and 5-year mortality in untreated patients is 50%.

Radiographically, these tumors are usually very small microadenomas. In some instances, they may not be visualized on neuroimaging, warranting empirical exploratory surgery. Measuring ACTH levels in the inferior petrosal sinus and using intraoperative ultrasound may help to localize the tumor. Resection is curative; most failures result from inability to find the tumor. Repeat surgery remains the treatment of choice for persistent Cushing disease. Other treatment options include radiotherapy, temporizing medical management and bilateral adrenalectomy.

TABLE 10.4

Hormonal basis for diagnosis of Cushing disease

- Elevated 24-hour urinary free cortisol
- Loss of ACTH suppression by glucocorticoids
- Elevated ACTH levels
- Exclusion of ectopic ACTH secretion

ACTH, adrenocorticotropic hormone

TABLE 10.5

Causes of ectopic ACTH secretion

- Small-cell lung cancer
- Carcinoid tumor
- Other tumors

In 10–15% of patients undergoing bilateral adrenalectomy, ACTH secretion persists or progresses, with accompanying enlargement of the sellar lesion, progressive neurological symptoms and secondary skin hyperpigmentation. This combination of features is known as Nelson syndrome. Further surgery and radiotherapy may control symptoms. However, 20% of patients die of complications or distant metastases.

TSH-secreting pituitary adenomas

TSH-secreting pituitary adenomas account for fewer than 1% of pituitary adenomas and are defined by persistent elevation of TSH in the setting of increased levels of circulating thyroxine and other thyroid hormones. Elevation of the glycoprotein α subunit in 80% of patients distinguishes these tumors from primary thyroiditis. A combination of surgery and radiotherapy is often necessary to control these tumors.

Gonadotropin-secreting pituitary adenomas

Gonadotropin-secreting pituitary adenomas account for 10–15% of all pituitary adenomas. Although they secrete FSH or luteinizing-stimulating hormone (LSH), most are endocrinologically asymptomatic and present with neurological symptoms related to compression. Most are macroadenomas and should be treated surgically.

Non-secreting pituitary adenomas

Approximately 25–30% of pituitary adenomas do not secrete any hormone and are most commonly categorized as null cell adenomas. Surgery is indicated to preserve or restore both neurological and endocrinological function, although it is reasonable to follow small, clinically silent, incidental pituitary adenomas clinically and radiographically.

Pituitary carcinomas

Pituitary carcinomas result from the rare situation in which a previously benign pituitary adenoma disseminates throughout the neuraxis or develops systemic metastasis. The diagnosis is predicated on evidence of metastasis (i.e. radiographic evidence of CNS dissemination or systemic tumor), as opposed to the usual histological criteria of malignancy. Most patients with a pituitary carcinoma previously had a secreting pituitary adenoma, and patients with Nelson syndrome are at greatest risk of developing a pituitary carcinoma.

The main treatment options are surgical resection and radiotherapy. Attempts to use chemotherapy have generally been disappointing, but medical management of secreting tumors may provide some palliation. The prognosis is generally poor, with a 1-year mortality in excess of 50%.

Craniopharyngiomas

Craniopharyngiomas are low-grade tumors that arise in the suprasellar region. They are thought to derive from remnants of Rathke pouch, the embryological precursor to the anterior pituitary gland, oral mucosa and teeth.

About half of all craniopharyngiomas occur in children and the other half in adults. Pathologically, these tumors are divided into the adamantinomatous type (calcified multicystic lesions that typically occur in children aged 5–9 years, and are rare in adults) and squamous papillary lesions (more often solid, occurring primarily in adults). Radiographically, 75% of these tumors will calcify; this, in combination with the characteristic MRI appearance, often helps to distinguish craniopharyngiomas from other lesions of the sellar region (Figure 10.3).

Clinically, craniopharyngiomas can present with a mix of neurological and endocrinological symptoms. In contrast to pituitary adenomas, craniopharyngiomas commonly cause diabetes insipidus. Children often present with growth failure, and adults with amenorrhea or impotence. Depending on their location, these tumors can cause compression of the optic chiasm, obstructive hydrocephalus or hypothalamic dysfunction.

Surgical resection is the treatment of choice. With current microscopic techniques, it is increasingly possible to achieve a gross total resection. However, these lesions are often contained by a pseudocapsule with additional rests of adherent tumor that may not be completely resected. Furthermore, the benefit of gross total resection

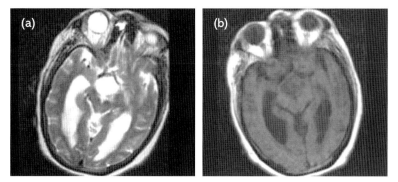

Figure 10.3 (a) Non-contrast axial T2-weighted and (b) non-contrast axial T1-weighted images of an adamantinomatous type craniopharyngioma in an 80-year-old woman. This patient presented primarily with behavioral changes and diabetes insipidus. The lesion demonstrated diffuse irregular contrast enhancement following gadolinium administration.

should be weighed against the risk of secondary neurological or endocrine dysfunction. Patients who have diabetes insipidus preoperatively are unlikely to improve, and those without the disorder have a moderate risk of surgically induced diabetes insipidus that may or may not be reversible.

The tumor recurs in approximately 25% of patients undergoing a gross total resection. The recurrence rate is higher for subtotal resection, but it nevertheless provides long-term control for 50% or more of patients.

Radiotherapy can be used for patients with recurrent or inoperable tumor. Stereotactic radiosurgery or direct interstitial radiotherapy may be appropriate for selected patients. Direct injection of bleomycin into recurrent tumoral cysts has been reported to prevent re-accumulation.

Key points – pituitary tumors

- Pituitary adenomas may present with endocrine or neurological abnormalities, or both.
- The goals of therapy include: reversal of endocrinopathy; elimination of mass effect with preservation or restoration of neurological function (particularly vision); prevention of recurrence.
- Patients with prolactinomas should be managed medically; most other pituitary adenomas require surgery, with or without radiotherapy.
- Endocrine consultation is critical in the initial assessment and ongoing management of all patients with pituitary region tumors (adenomas, craniopharyngiomas and germ cell tumors).

Key references

Cannavo S, Curto L, Squadrito S et al. Cabergoline: a first-choice treatment in patients with previously untreated prolactin-secreting pituitary adenoma. *J Endocrinol Invest* 1999;22:354–9.

Merchant TE, Kiehna EN, Sanford RA et al. Craniopharyngioma: the St Jude Children's Research Hospital experience 1984–2001. *Int J Radiat Oncol Biol Phys* 2002;53:533–42.

Reitmeyer M, Vance ML, Laws ER. The neurosurgical management of Cushing's disease. *Mol Cell Endocrinol* 2002;197:73–9.

Tyrrell JB, Lamborn KR, Hannegan LT et al. Transsphenoidal microsurgical therapy of prolactinomas: initial outcomes and long-term results. *Neurosurgery* 1999;44:254–61, discussion 261–3.

Van Effenterre R, Boch AL. Craniopharyngioma in adults and children: a study of 122 surgical cases. *J Neurosurg* 2002;97:3–11.

Primary central nervous system lymphoma (PCNSL) is a rare form of non-Hodgkin lymphoma confined to the CNS. This tumor is of interest for several reasons. First, it has increased in incidence in immunocompetent patients over the past few decades. This increase is independent of advances in neuroimaging or the general aging of the population. Therefore, it is an increasingly important consideration in the differential diagnosis of intracranial mass lesions. Second, unlike many primary brain tumors, PCNSL is exquisitely responsive to treatment and aggressive management may lead to prolonged remission or cure. Finally, the long-term consequences of aggressive therapy may cause significant delayed neurological toxicity.

Etiology

There is no known etiology or risk factor for the development of PCNSL in the immunocompetent patient. Human herpesvirus 6 and 8, as well as Epstein-Barr virus, have been evaluated without evidence of any association. Clonal abnormalities of chromosomes 1, 6, 7 and 14, identical to those detected in systemic non-Hodgkin lymphoma, have been found in PCNSL. Analysis of cell surface markers, including neural cell adhesion molecule (NCAM) and integrins, are also identical to those found in systemic lymphoma. In addition, p15 and p16 deletions have been described.

Pathology

Histologically, PCNSL is indistinguishable from systemic non-Hodgkin lymphoma. At least 90% of cases are B-cell lymphomas (CD20+) of the diffuse large cell, large cell immunoblastic or lymphoblastic type. Microscopically, PCNSL is a diffuse lesion with a characteristic angiocentric growth pattern; some tumors may even invade the blood vessel wall. Autopsy studies have demonstrated widespread infiltration of malignant lymphocytes into normal brain. Small, benign, reactive

T-lymphocytes infiltrate throughout the tumor and reactive astrocytes are common.

Clinical features and evaluation

The typical patient is in the age range 55–70 years, and most have had symptoms for only a few weeks before seeking medical attention. Cognitive and personality changes are the most common initial symptoms, reflecting involvement of the frontal lobes, corpus callosum and deep periventricular structures. PCNSL is often multifocal and may present with any focal neurological finding, such as hemiparesis or aphasia. Seizures are a presenting complaint in only about 10% of cases, which is less common than in patients with glioma or brain metastasis. The most important prognostic factors are age less than 60 years and an excellent performance status.

Evidence of leptomeningeal dissemination is found in up to 40% of patients, but concomitant clinical findings are uncommon. Therefore, CSF should be obtained from all newly diagnosed patients, and analyzed for cell count, protein, glucose and cytology. Tumor markers (including lactate dehydrogenase isoenzymes, β-glucuronidase and β2-microglobulin), immunocytochemical analysis and polymerase chain reaction (PCR) detection of immunoglobulin gene rearrangements may be useful if CSF cytology is negative or inconclusive. Primary leptomeningeal lymphoma is rare and usually presents with signs and symptoms of increased intracranial pressure, multifocal cranial neuropathies or nerve root involvement.

About 15% of patients with PCNSL have ocular involvement, and 50–80% of those with isolated ocular lymphoma develop parenchymal brain lymphoma. Symptoms include blurred, cloudy vision, decreased visual acuity or 'floaters', but many patients are asymptomatic. Complete ophthalmologic evaluation, including slit lamp examination, is recommended in all newly diagnosed patients.

Systemic lymphoma is an uncommon finding (occurring in 3–5% of PCNSL patients) and the need to perform a comprehensive assessment of the systemic extent of disease is controversial. The standard modalities used to evaluate systemic disease are CT scanning of the chest, abdomen and pelvis, and bone marrow biopsy. There is also increasing use of 18-fluoro-2-deoxyglucose PET.

Gadolinium-enhanced MRI is the standard neuroimaging technique for the evaluation of PCNSL. Most lesions are supratentorial and periventricular, often involving deep structures such as the corpus callosum and basal ganglia. Lesions may be hypointense or hyperintense on pre-contrast T1 imaging, with dense, homogeneous enhancement after the administration of gadolinium. Peritumoral edema and local mass effect are often less than expected with other intracranial lesions. Calcification, hemorrhage or cyst formation are rare.

Table 11.1 summarizes the approaches to evaluating patients with newly diagnosed PCNSL. Ideally, all patients with newly diagnosed PCNSL should be treated as part of a clinical trial or referred to an appropriate tertiary care center for evaluation and treatment.

Differential diagnosis

The main differential diagnosis is malignant glioma. Multifocal lesions raise the possibility of metastatic disease, and this may be confounded by the fact that as many as 15% of PCNSL patients have a previous diagnosis of systemic cancer. The exquisite sensitivity of PCNSL to corticosteroids may lead to consideration of multiple sclerosis or neurosarcoidosis as possible diagnoses.

TABLE 11.1

Evaluation of newly diagnosed PCNSL

- MRI of the brain with gadolinium
- CSF cytology
- Ophthalmologic evaluation with slit lamp examination
- Bone marrow biopsy
- CT of the chest, abdomen and pelvis
- Consider MRI of the spine with gadolinium, if symptomatic

Treatment

Surgery is performed to allow a histopathologic diagnosis to be reached. Stereotactic needle biopsy is the procedure of choice. In contrast to most other primary brain tumors, aggressive resection does not improve survival and may result in neurological deterioration.

Corticosteroids are used in the treatment of vasogenic edema caused by intracranial tumors. In PCNSL, corticosteroids also have a potent oncolytic effect, causing tumor cell lysis and radiographic regression in up to 40% of patients. The onset of action is rapid, with resolution of symptoms and marked reduction in tumor size within 24–48 hours. Therefore, steroids should be withheld in any patient with a presumptive diagnosis of PCNSL until histopathologic diagnosis is secured.

Radiotherapy. PCNSL is a radiosensitive tumor and whole-brain radiotherapy was the standard treatment for many years. Median survival with radiotherapy is 10–18 months; with corticosteroids alone the figure is 6–8 weeks. Although microscopic CSF dissemination is common, more extensive craniospinal radiotherapy does not confer additional survival benefit and is associated with significant morbidity, which limits the use of adjuvant chemotherapy.

The optimal dose of whole-brain radiotherapy is 40–50 Gy. Doses greater than 50 Gy have been associated with an increased risk of delayed neurotoxicity. The addition of a focal boost does not improve local tumor control or survival. Ongoing studies are examining the role of hyperfractionated radiotherapy, as well as lower doses of radiotherapy in chemosensitive patients.

In patients with ocular lymphoma, the posterior two-thirds of the globe should be irradiated to a dose of 36–40 Gy. Recurrent visual symptoms may represent recurrent ocular lymphoma or secondary radiotherapy-related toxicity, such as epithelioid keratopathy, posterior cataracts, retinopathy or optic neuropathy.

Chemotherapy. PCNSL is a chemosensitive tumor. However, the standard agents used in the treatment of non-Hodgkin lymphoma are not effective, because they are unable to penetrate the blood–brain barrier. High-dose methotrexate is the single most effective agent in the treatment of PCNSL (Figure 11.1). Doses of 1 g/m^2 or more result in tumoricidal levels in the brain, and doses of 3.5 g/m^2 or more yield tumoricidal levels in the CSF. Therefore, most treatment regimens incorporate high-dose methotrexate (1–8 g/m^2) alone or in combination with other chemotherapeutic agents, followed by whole-brain radiotherapy. This combined modality approach has resulted in

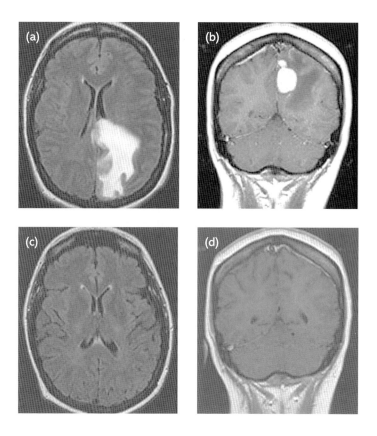

Figure 11.1 (a) Axial FLAIR and (b) gadolinium-enhanced T1-weighted coronal images of a 45-year-old woman with PCNSL before chemotherapy. (c) and (d) Corresponding scans after five cycles of high-dose methotrexate in combination with procarbazine and vincristine demonstrate complete resolution of the tumor.

response rates in excess of 75% and median survival in the range 30–60 months.

There has been increasing interest in using chemotherapy alone in order to minimize delayed neurological toxicity. In older patients (≥ 60 years), methotrexate-based chemotherapy alone can achieve similar overall survival to that achieved with combined modality treatment. Importantly, older patients are able to tolerate aggressive chemotherapy without any excess acute morbidity. Typically, these patients improve during the course of chemotherapy, with resolution of neurocognitive deficits and improved performance status.

Relapse

The risk of relapse following the best current therapy is about 50%. Most recurrences are seen within 2 years of diagnosis, but late relapses have been reported. Extent of disease at diagnosis may be an important determinant for risk of relapse, with ocular or leptomeningeal disease conferring a higher likelihood of recurrence. Parenchymal brain relapse, either at the primary site or a distant site within the brain, is most frequent (Figure 11.2); however, CSF and leptomeningeal relapses are seen and systemic relapse may be as high as 10%.

The prognosis at relapse is generally poor. However, prolonged survival is possible and some patients continue to be sensitive to salvage

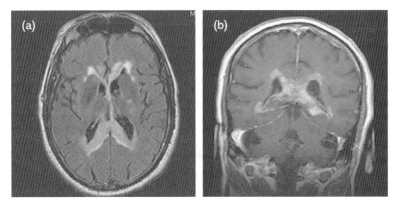

Figure 11.2 (a) Axial FLAIR and (b) gadolinium-enhanced T1-weighted coronal images of a 74-year-old man with recurrent PCNSL replacing the majority of the corpus callosum.

therapy despite multiple relapses. There is no standard salvage therapy. Success has been reported using methotrexate (even in patients previously treated with methotrexate), high-dose cytarabine, PCV (procarbazine, lomustine and vincristine), temozolomide and rituximab. Radiotherapy is particularly effective for ocular relapse. Older patients who defer initial radiotherapy remain responsive to this treatment modality, but are at high risk of developing subsequent neurotoxicity.

Treatment-related neurotoxicity

Delayed neurological toxicity is increasingly recognized in long-term PCNSL survivors who were treated with methotrexate followed by cranial radiotherapy. The risk is greatest in older patients; of those aged over 60 years who survive 1 year, up to 90% are affected. The average patient becomes symptomatic within months of treatment and has a significant decline in performance status, necessitating constant supervision and care.

The clinical syndrome of delayed neurological toxicity is characterized by a triad of dementia, gait ataxia and urinary dysfunction (Figure 11.3). A diagnosis of delayed neurotoxicity requires

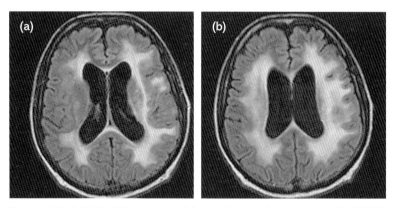

Figure 11.3 Axial FLAIR images of a 54-year-old man who was treated for PCNSL 4 years previously. These images demonstrate large confluent areas of abnormality consistent with a leukoencephalopathy. The patient went into an abrupt symptomatic decline around the time these images were obtained, with cognitive dysfunction, ataxia and incontinence. Placement of a ventriculoperitoneal shunt achieved a modest improvement. There was no evidence of recurrent tumor.

exclusion of recurrent PCNSL by neuroimaging and CSF cytology. Radiographic and pathological findings are most consistent with a leukoencephalopathy. Attempts to treat delayed neurotoxicity have been generally unrewarding, although a few patients may have transient improvement following placement of a ventriculoperitoneal shunt. Other agents, such as methylphenidate, have been successful in individual patients.

Delayed treatment-related cerebrovascular disease has been observed in younger patients 7–10 years after completion of therapy. This may occur alone or in conjunction with a progressive leukoencephalopathy. Accelerated atherosclerosis is a known complication of cranial radiotherapy that typically develops 10–20 years after treatment. PCNSL may further predispose to cerebrovascular damage if lysis of angiocentric tumor cells damages neighboring endothelium.

HIV-related PCNSL

PCNSL occurs in 1.6–9.0% of the HIV-infected population and is the second most common intracranial mass lesion in this group of patients, after toxoplasmosis. Before the introduction of highly active antiretroviral therapy (HAART), the incidence of PCNSL in the HIV-infected population was continuing to rise. However, there has since been a significant decline in HIV-related PCNSL.

HIV-related PCNSL is associated with infection of B-lymphocytes by Epstein-Barr virus. After a primary Epstein-Barr viral infection, latently infected lymphocytes persist for the remainder of a person's life. Immunosuppression with an attendant decrease in suppressor T-cell function allows uncontrolled proliferation of the immortalized latently infected lymphocytes, with subsequent development of a neoplasm. There is a propensity for the lymphoma to develop in the CNS of these patients, presumably because of decreased immune surveillance.

Patients with HIV-related PCNSL have a median age of 30–40 years and seizures are a more common presenting feature than in other PCNSL patients (encountered in 25% of cases). The median latency from the time of diagnosis of HIV infection is approximately 5 years, and the development of PCNSL is often associated with the onset of other HIV-related diseases. Some studies have found a higher incidence of multiple lesions in HIV-related PCNSL; however, multifocal lesions in AIDS patients may have multiple concurrent etiologies.

The major differential diagnosis is toxoplasmosis. Although patterns of CNS disease in AIDS patients have been changing, toxoplasmosis and PCNSL remain the most common intracranial lesions. Improved therapeutic options and prolonged survival in HIV-positive patients mandate an aggressive approach to achieving a precise diagnosis for an intracranial lesion. SPECT or PET may be useful in differentiating between PCNSL and infectious processes. Thallium-201 SPECT scanning, when positive, is highly specific for PCNSL; similar results have been obtained with 18-fluoro-2-deoxyglucose PET. The specificity of SPECT may be further enhanced with delayed imaging and calculation of the thallium retention index.

The identification of Epstein-Barr viral DNA in the CSF strongly suggests a diagnosis of PCNSL. The combined results of thallium-201 SPECT and Epstein-Barr viral DNA testing eliminate the need for a brain biopsy in many patients with AIDS . However, if the diagnosis remains unclear, a diagnostic biopsy should be performed.

Treatment is influenced by the clinical assessment of the patient. Patients in good condition may benefit from aggressive combined modality therapy, which confers a median survival in the range of 3–19 months. However, many patients are not able to tolerate this approach. Those treated with conventional radiotherapy and corticosteroids have a median survival of 2–5 months. Initiation of HAART has been reported to result in remission.

Ocular lymphoma

Ocular lymphoma, a variant of PCNSL, is also increasing in incidence. Unlike cerebral PCNSL, diagnosis is often delayed and a misdiagnosis of chronic vitreitis or uveitis is common. Careful slit lamp examination and vitrectomy are essential for making a definitive diagnosis.

The best treatment option for this subset of patients is aggressive combined modality treatment incorporating ocular radiotherapy and systemic chemotherapy. Direct administration of intraocular chemotherapy is being studied. Patients treated for isolated ocular lymphoma have an 80% risk of developing cerebral involvement as long as 10 years after initial diagnosis. Therefore, meticulous long-term follow-up is mandatory.

Key points

- PCNSL is increasing in incidence in the immunocompetent population.
- The approach to diagnosis and treatment of PCNSL is significantly different from other primary brain tumors:
  - steroids should be avoided prior to obtaining diagnostic tissue
  - stereotactic biopsy should be used for tissue diagnosis; complete resection is not indicated
  - optimal treatment includes methotrexate-based chemotherapy, with or without cranial radiotherapy
  - older patients should be treated with chemotherapy alone to avoid treatment-related dementia.
- Ideally, all patients with newly diagnosed PCNSL should be treated as part of a clinical trial or referred to an appropriate tertiary care center for evaluation and treatment.

Key references

Abrey LE, Yahalom J, DeAngelis LM. Treatment for primary CNS lymphoma: the next step. *J Clin Oncol* 2000;18:3144–50.

DeAngelis LM, Seiferheld W, Schold SC et al. Combination chemotherapy and radiotherapy for primary central nervous system lymphoma: Radiation Therapy Oncology Group Study 93-10. *J Clin Oncol* 2002;20: 4643–8.

Doolittle ND, Miner ME, Hall WA et al. Safety and efficacy of a multicenter study using intraarterial chemotherapy in conjunction with osmotic opening of the blood–brain barrier for the treatment of patients with malignant brain tumors. *Cancer* 2000;88:637–47.

Ferreri AJ, Blay JY, Reni M et al. Prognostic scoring system for primary CNS lymphomas: the international extranodal lymphoma study group experience. *J Clin Oncol* 2003;21:266–72.

Olson JE, Janney CA, Rao RD et al. The continuing increase in the incidence of primary central nervous system non-Hodgkin lymphoma: a surveillance, epidemiology, and end results analysis. *Cancer* 2002;95:1504–10.

Soussain C, Suzan F, Hoang-Xuan K et al. Results of intensive chemotherapy followed by hematopoietic stem-cell rescue in 22 patients with refractory or recurrent primary CNS lymphoma or intraocular lymphoma. *J Clin Oncol* 2001;19:742–9.

The vast majority of primary brain tumors occur sporadically, but a small number appear to be familial. The etiology of sporadic brain tumors is unknown, but environmental factors are suspected. Most patients with a family history of primary brain tumors have a hereditary disease that is known to be associated with such tumors, such as tuberous sclerosis, neurofibromatosis, familial polyposis or Li–Fraumeni syndrome. However, some patients do not have any underlying or obvious hereditary disorder that would predispose them to primary brain tumors, but nevertheless give a striking history of these tumors in first-degree relatives. Usually, the tumors are found to be high-grade gliomas.

Although it is feasible that germline abnormalities could lead to the development of primary brain tumors in these families, there are a number of unusual demographic features suggesting an environmental rather than genetic explanation for brain tumor clustering. Most cases of confirmed familial cancers are multigenerational, and affected individuals are younger than average for the tumor. However, brain tumor families who do not have one of the recognized hereditary diseases usually involve parent–child and sibling–sibling cases; it is rare for more than two generations to be involved. In addition, the demographics suggest environmental rather than genetic causes in the parent–child and sibling–sibling clusters. These observations suggest that familial exposure to an environmental toxin or ionizing radiation may account for the clustering of primary brain tumors in these families.

It is important for clinicians to enquire about any family history of brain tumors, and to be aware of the major syndromes with neoplastic manifestations in the nervous system, so that these diagnoses are not missed. Recognizing a familial brain tumor syndrome is valuable for appropriate patient surveillance for another occult brain tumor or associated disease, for screening family members, and for genetic counseling. Most patients presenting with primary brain tumors will, however, be sporadic cases and the etiology will remain unknown.

Neurofibromatosis type 1

Neurofibromatosis type 1 is an autosomal dominant disorder with an estimated incidence of 1/4000. The gene responsible for this disorder, NF1, is located on chromosome 17q12. Diagnosis requires the presence of two or more of the following features:

- six or more café au lait spots
- two or more neurofibromas or one plexiform neurofibroma
- axillary or inguinal freckling
- optic nerve glioma
- characteristic osseous lesions
- a first-degree relative with neurofibromatosis type 1.

The major neoplastic neurological manifestations of this disorder are optic nerve glioma, astrocytoma and glioblastoma multiforme. The main non-neoplastic neurological features are seizures, cognitive impairment and hydrocephalus (Figure 12.1).

Neurofibromatosis type 2

Neurofibromatosis type 2 is an autosomal dominant disorder with an estimated incidence of 1/40 000. The gene responsible for this disorder, NF2, is located on 22q12. For a diagnosis of neurofibromatosis type 2 to be made, specific features must be identified:

- bilateral vestibular hamartomas, *or*

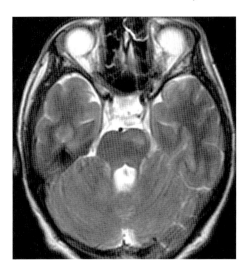

Figure 12.1 T2-weighted axial MRI of a 26-year-old woman with neurofibromatosis type 1, demonstrating a non-enhancing optic chiasm glioma.

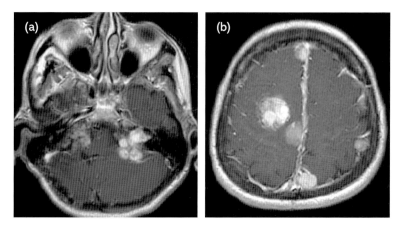

Figure 12.2 T2-weighted axial MRI of a 47-year-old woman with neurofibromatosis type 2 demonstrating: (a) bilateral acoustic nerve schwannomas; (b) multiple meningiomas.

- a first-degree relative with neurofibromatosis type 2, in combination either with a unilateral vestibular schwannoma or with at least two of the following: meningioma, glioma, schwannoma, neurofibroma, posterior subcapsular lens opacity or cerebral calcification, *or*
- two of the following:
  - unilateral vestibular schwannoma
  - multiple meningiomas
  - any one of schwannoma, neurofibroma, glioma, posterior subcapsular lens opacity or cerebral calcification.

The major neoplastic neurological manifestations are schwannoma, meningioma, astrocytoma, ependymoma and glial hamartoma, while the principal non-neoplastic neurological manifestation is cerebral calcifications (Figure 12.2)

Von Hippel–Lindau disease

Von Hippel–Lindau disease is an autosomal dominant disorder and is extremely rare. The gene responsible for this disease is located on 3p25-26. The diagnostic criteria are:

- capillary hemangioblastoma in the central nervous system or retina, *and either*

- one of the following tumors: renal cell carcinoma, pancreatic adenomas or islet cell tumors, pheochromocytomas, epididymal cystadenomas or endolymphatic sac tumor, *or*
- a first-degree relative with Von Hippel–Lindau disease.

The major neoplastic neurological manifestation is hemangioblastoma of the central nervous system; there are no non-neoplastic neurological manifestations (Figure 12.3).

Tuberous sclerosis

Tuberous sclerosis is a group of autosomal dominant disorders, with an incidence between 1/5000 and 1/10 000. The diagnostic criteria for tuberous sclerosis are:

- presence of hamartomas involving the skin, nervous system, retina, heart and kidneys (definite criterion)
- multiple cutaneous angiofibromas (probable criterion).

Neoplastic neurological manifestations include subependymal giant cell astrocytoma and retinal giant cell astrocytoma. Non-neoplastic neurological features are subependymal nodule, cortical tuber, white matter hamartoma and retinal hamartoma.

Li–Fraumeni syndrome

Li–Fraumeni syndrome is an autosomal dominant disorder in which there is an increased risk of multiple tumors developing in children and

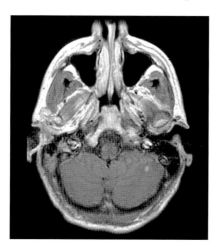

Figure 12.3 Contrast-enhanced axial MRI of a 23-year-old man with von Hippel–Lindau syndrome, demonstrating a small enhancing cerebellar nodule consistent with a cerebellar hemangioblastoma. The patient presented acutely with paraparesis following rupture of a spinal cord hemangioblastoma.

young adults, including breast cancer, soft-tissue sarcomas, osteosarcomas and primary brain tumors. The incidence of the disorder has not been established, but it is known to be due to a germline mutation of *TP53* on 17p13.

The diagnostic criteria are:
- occurrence of a sarcoma before the age of 45 years, *and either*
- at least one first-degree relative with any tumor before age 45, *or*
- a second- or first-degree relative with cancer before the age of 45 or a sarcoma at any age.

Neoplastic neurological manifestations of the disease are glioblastoma multiforme, anaplastic astrocytoma, low-grade astrocytoma, oligoastrocytoma, medulloblastoma and primitive neuroectodermal tumor. There are no non-neoplastic manifestations.

Turcot syndrome

Turcot syndrome comprises a group of autosomal dominant, and possibly also recessive, disorders characterized by multiple colorectal neoplasms and malignant neuroepithelial tumors. Multiple genes are implicated, including *APC* on 5q21, *hMLH1* on 3p21.3, and *hPMS2* on 7p22. The incidence of this syndrome is unknown.

Diagnosis requires the coexistence of primary brain and colon tumors. There are two distinct syndromes:
- medulloblastomas arising in the setting of familial adenomatous polyposis and involving germline mutations of *APC* gene
- glioblastoma multiforme arising in the setting of hereditary non-polyposis colorectal carcinoma and involving mutations of DNA mismatch repair genes *hMLH1* and *hPMS2*.

The neoplastic neurological manifestations of the syndrome are glioblastoma multiforme and medulloblastoma, and there are no non-neoplastic manifestations.

Key points – familial brain tumor syndromes

* There are several syndromes associated with an inherited predisposition to a variety of brain tumors. However, the vast majority of brain tumors are not inherited.
* Recognizing a familial brain tumor syndrome is valuable for appropriate surveillance of individuals at high risk of developing an occult brain tumor or associated disease and for genetic counseling.

Key references

Blatt J, Jaffee M, Deutsch M, Adkins JC. Neurofibromatosis and childhood tumors. *Cancer* 1986;57: 1225–9.

Chow CW, Klug GL, Lewis EA. Subependymal giant-cell astrocytoma in children. *J Neurosurg* 1988;68: 880–3.

Filling-Katz MR, Choyke PL, Oldfield E et al. Central nervous system involvement in von Hippel–Lindau disease. *Neurology* 1991;41:41–6.

Hamilton SR, Liu B, Parsons RE et al. The molecular basis of Turcot's syndrome. *N Engl J Med* 1995; 332:839–47.

Huson SM, Harper PS, Hourihan MD et al. Cerebellar haemangioblastoma and von Hippel-Lindau disease. *Brain* 1986;109:1297–1310.

Kanter WR, Eldridge R, Fabricant R et al. Central neurofibromatosis with bilateral acoustic neuroma: genetic, clinical and biochemical distinctions from peripheral neurofibromatosis. *Neurology* 1980;30:851–9.

Martuza RL, Ojemann RG. Bilateral acoustic neuromas: clinical aspects, pathogenesis, and treatment. *Neurosurgery* 1982;10:1–12.

Ponz de Leon M. Li–Fraumeni syndrome. Recent results. *Cancer Res* 1994;136:275–86.

Riccardi VM. Von Recklinghausen neurofibromatosis. *N Engl J Med* 1981;305:1617–26.

Several types of lesion may be mistaken for a primary intracranial tumor and must therefore be considered in the differential diagnosis of suggestive MRI abnormalities. These lesions often are cystic in nature, hence the greatest need for differentiation is from cystic tumors (Table 13.1).

Dermoid and epidermoid

Dermoids and epidermoids account for about 1% of intracranial tumors and are most often found at the base of the brain, fourth ventricle or spine. They are midline tumors that arise from fetal neural and ectodermal tissues. There may be direct communication with the skin via a midline dermal tract.

In addition to the typical midline location, epidermoids may arise in the lateral skull, cerebellopontine angle or ear (cholesteatoma). They present more often in adults than children, and are 3–4 times more common than dermoids. They consist primarily of a keratinized squamous epithelium (Figure 13.1).

TABLE 13.1

Differential diagnosis of a cystic MRI lesion

Tumors	Other lesions
• Pilocytic astrocytoma	• Colloid cyst of the third ventricle
• Ganglion cell tumors	
• Ependymoma	• Rathke cleft cyst
• Hemangioblastoma	• Endodermal cyst
• Pleomorphic xanthoastrocytoma	• Choroid plexus cyst
	• Epidermoid
• Craniopharyngioma	• Dermoid
	• Arachnoid cyst
	• Pineal cyst

Dermoids are distinguished from epidermoids by the presence of dermal appendages (hair, teeth, adnexa and fat) in addition to keratinized squamous epithelium (Figure 13.2). They are more likely to have a dermal sinus tract. These lesions typically present in childhood.

Both types of lesion slowly expand as a result of epithelial turnover; dermoids may expand more rapidly as a result of secretions. Symptoms may arise secondary to mass effect or, in some cases, spontaneous rupture or leakage may result in aseptic meningitis. Patients who have recurrent aseptic meningitis should therefore be evaluated for a dermoid or epidermoid.

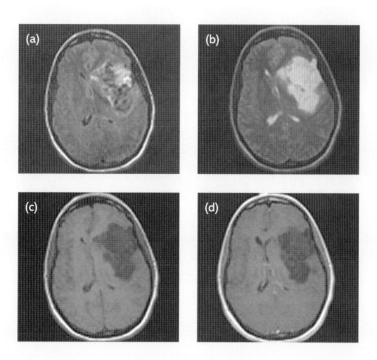

Figure 13.1 Multiple axial magnetic resonance images of an epidermoid of the temporal lobe in a 35-year-old woman presenting with seizures. (a) Mixed signal characteristics of FLAIR imaging and (b) high signal on T2-weighted imaging, that are typical of this tumor. (c) T1-weighted images without and (d) with contrast demonstrate low signal and lack of contrast enhancement.

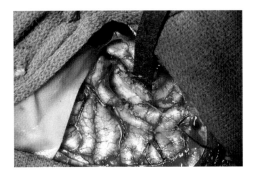

Figure 13.2 Intraoperative photograph of a dermoid cyst, showing the typical yellowish appearance that results from the high lipid content often found in these cysts.

Treatment is resection. Intraoperative leakage of cyst contents may cause cranial neuropathies, aseptic meningitis or secondary hydrocephalus due to obstruction of arachnoid granulations. Complete resection may be more difficult to achieve for epidermoids than for dermoids. Subtotal resection is appropriate when total resection is not feasible.

Colloid cyst of the third ventricle

Colloid cysts of the third ventricle are sessile masses attached to the choroid plexus at the foramen of Munro (Figure 13.3). They cause obstructive hydrocephalus, which often presents with intermittent symptoms attributed to transient increases in intracranial pressure, referred to as 'plateau waves'.

Previously, these lesions were thought to cause intermittent symptoms by a ball-valve mechanism that caused intermittent obstruction of the foramen of Munro with changes in posture. However, it is now known that the attachment to the choroid plexus is fixed and does not move.

Patients who are experiencing symptoms should have the cyst resected; often, an endoscopic approach is used to achieve safe removal. Ventriculoperitoneal shunts are best avoided in these patients; both lateral ventricles may require independent shunting and obstruction rates are high. It is safe to follow asymptomatic patients radiographically.

Rathke cleft cyst

Rathke cleft cysts are usually small asymptomatic abnormalities found on MRI. They can arise in either the sellar or suprasellar

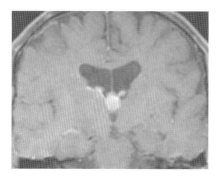

Figure 13.3 Gadolinium-enhanced T1-weighted coronal image of a colloid cyst of the third ventricle.

region, with 70% of these cysts bridging these two compartments. The lack of calcification may help to distinguish these cysts from craniopharyngiomas. Rarely, Rathke cleft cysts cause pituitary dysfunction, headache or visual disturbance; in these cases, surgical resection is appropriate. Recurrence is rare.

Arachnoid cyst

Arachnoid cysts are congenital malformations that are typically found in a superficial location, but may be intraventricular (Figure 13.4). They are usually asymptomatic, but occasionally have sufficient mass effect to cause headaches or seizures. Symptomatic lesions should be surgically drained.

Neurenteric cyst

Neurenteric cysts are congenital epithelial cysts that occur in the spinal canal or posterior fossa. Most are asymptomatic; those causing compression or obstruction of CSF flow should be resected or diverted.

Key points

- Dermoids and epidermoids are benign congenital lesions that typically produce symptoms as they gradually increase in size.
- Total or subtotal resection is the treatment of choice for dermoids and epidermoids.
- Colloid cysts should be resected using modern microneurosurgical techniques.

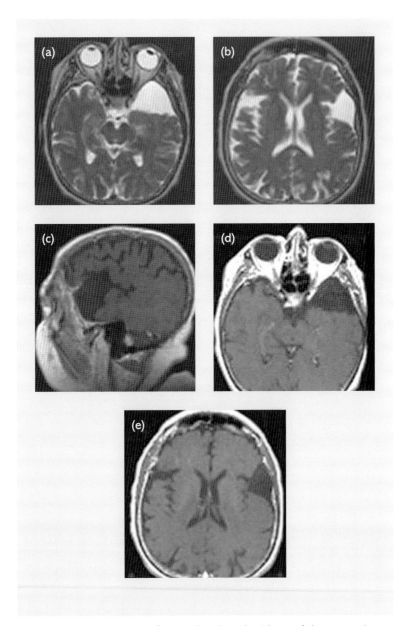

Figure 13.4 Multiple images of an incidental arachnoid cyst of the temporal lobe, the most common location of these cysts. The contents of the cyst have a similar appearance to CSF on both T2-weighted images (a and b) and T1-weighted images (c, d and e).

Key references

Cobbs CS, Pitts LH, Wilson CB. Epidermoid and dermoid cysts of the posterior fossa. *Clin Neurosurg* 1997;44:511–28.

Desai KI, Nadkarni TD, Muzumdar DP, Goel AH. Surgical management of colloid cyst of the third ventricle – a study of 105 cases. *Surg Neurol* 2002;57:295–302, discussion 302–4.

Mathiesen T, Grane P, Lindgren L, Lindquist C. Third ventricle colloid cysts: a consecutive 12-year series. *J Neurosurg* 1997;86:5–12.

Sano K. Intracranial dysembryogenetic tumors: pathogenesis and their order of malignancy. *Neurosurg Rev* 2001;24:162–7, discussion 168–70.

Yasargil MG, Abernathy CD, Sarioglu AC. Microneurosurgical treatment of intracranial dermoid and epidermoid tumors. *Neurosurgery* 1989;24:561–7.

The management of brain tumors remains a major challenge because most cancers that involve the central nervous system remain incurable. However, brain tumors are a focus of intensive clinical investigation. Advances in our understanding of the molecular events underpinning tumor development, active drug discovery programs fostered by large pharmaceutical enterprises, and technological advances in neuroimaging will lead to changes in how clinicians manage brain tumors. Ultimately, this will result in an improved prognosis for patients suffering from these devastating illnesses.

Over the past decade, several key molecular events in tumor development have been identified. For instance, genetic changes leading to the formation of gliomas appear to involve two cellular functions: growth factor signaling and cell cycle control. Moreover, a number of successive genetic aberrations are required to transform an astrocyte into a cancerous cell, and there are a variety of apparently distinct genetic pathways leading to the formation of a malignant glioma such as a glioblastoma multiforme.

These recent discoveries have several significant implications. First, the genetic profile of a tumor can be used to establish an accurate neuropathological diagnosis. For example, the diagnosis of an anaplastic oligodendroglioma has traditionally been a difficult one, in part because of the variable histological appearance of this neoplasm and the absence of a reliable and specific immunohistochemical marker. However, loss of the short arm of chromosome 1 and the long arm of chromosome 19 have now been linked to a major subset of anaplastic oligodendrogliomas that are predictably chemosensitive and associated with a favorable prognosis. Thus, these changes can be used to establish a genetic diagnosis that is useful both for guiding therapy and for counseling patients. Ongoing research efforts will identify new markers that serve similar roles for other brain tumors, including glioblastoma, where there is already evidence of several distinct genetic subsets.

Second, advances in neuroimaging are likely to capitalize on these developments. Conventional neuroimaging for brain tumors consists of

MRI and PET. Magnetic resonance spectroscopy is a procedure that is similar to MRI, except that biochemical spectra of significance to brain tumors are measured. The spectral pattern can help identify the type and grade of tumor, and distinguish tumors from other disorders such as demyelination and infections. At present, this technology is experimental and not entirely accurate and reliable.

Other advances in neuroimaging involve the use of molecular probes targeted at specific genetic abnormalities, such as growth factor receptor upregulation, oncogene activation or tumor suppressor gene inactivation, to provide molecular images of brain tumors. This exciting field draws inspiration from advances in molecular biology and holds great promise not only for providing accurate non-invasive diagnosis of brain tumors, but also for guiding therapy based on specific molecular characteristics of a given tumor.

Third, the elucidation of critical or significant genetic alterations important for tumor formation and progression may identify therapeutic targets for drug development. Overexpression of platelet-derived growth factor and receptor, and epidermal growth factor receptor appear to be important events in many primary astrocytomas. The recent development of a variety of classes of novel drugs that antagonize these receptors, or disrupt downstream signaling pathways coupled to these receptors, offers the possibility of effective therapeutic approaches to these diseases. Similar agents are being developed that interfere with tumor angiogenesis and cell cycle control. Thus, future drug development for primary brain tumors is likely to be intimately linked to advances in our understanding of molecular carcinogenesis.

Ultimately, molecular characterization of a brain tumor will not only provide an accurate pathological diagnosis, but will also identify a rational therapeutic approach based on the unique genetic signature of the patient's tumor.

Useful addresses

American Brain Tumor Association
2720 River Road
Des Plaines, IL 60018
Tel: 847 827 9910
Fax: 847 827 9918
Patient line: 800 886 2282
info@abta.org
http://www.abta.org

National Brain Tumor Foundation
414 Thirteenth Street, Suite 700
Oakland, CA 94612-2603
Tel: 510 839 9777
Fax: 510 839 9779
nbtf@braintumor.org
http://www.braintumor.org
Brain Tumor Information Line:
1 800 934 CURE (2873)

National Cancer Institute
Brain tumor homepage
http://cancer.gov/cancerinfo/types/brain

The Society for Neuro-Oncology
http://www.soc-neuro-onc.org

Index